107

Rotator Cuff Exercises

TO BUILD, PROTECT AND MAINTAIN A HEALTHY
ROTATOR CUFF FOR LIFE

BY

ZACH CALHOON

Disclaimer

The material provided in this eBook are designed for informational and educational purposes only. The information in this book or any website associated with this book is not engaged in rendering medical advice or recommendation. You should not rely on any information in this book or from this website, including but not limited to meal plans, fitness programs, information in text files, messages, or articles on this page to replace consultations with qualified health care professionals to meet your individual medical needs. Information accessible on this site www.rubberarmseries.com is not intended to be a substitute for professional medical advice. Some information in our material will help some and not others. Depending upon your needs and situation, you may have an completely different experience with the rubberarmseries.com . Individuals should never disregard professional medical advice or delay in seeking it because of something they read, heard, or watched on rubberarmseries.com or their eBook or program material. We at rubberarmseries.com strongly recommend that all individuals seek advice from their general practitioner, doctor, dietician, nutritionist or professional before taking part on any diet or exercise plan shown on our website, information or products offered. We at rubberarmseries.com take no responsibility for use of misuse of products purchased from rubberarmseries.com or anything written or said by Zach Calhoon. By participating in any diet or exercise plan on this site or in this eBook you acknowledge that you may injure yourself as a result of participation and agree to hereby release owners/directors of www.rubberarmseries.com from any liability including, but not limited to muscle pulls, muscle sprains, broken bones, heart attacks, stroke, diabetes, related incidents, shin splints, other orthopedic related injuries, gout, soreness, and any other health-related incident during participation. Purchase of any product from rubberarmseries.com would in action, agreement with these terms. By purchase of any product from rubberarmseries.com you acknowledge that you, or an additional party, will never sue this site or owner of this site.

TABLE OF CONTENTS

INTRODUCTION

How's your shoulder doing?

Do you have any pain? Do you lack range of motion? Or do you just experience some occasional soreness?

Many people have shoulder problems. Soreness, weakness and pain. It's a common problem (Especially for overhead athletes). You can still function and live "ok" with a underperforming shoulder. Most shoulder problems (and weakness) are ignored.

Over time, your shoulder weakness, starts to cause more and more problems. Then one day, boom you have a tear. Hello surgery, recovery and physically therapy.

This sequence is so common, and holds your back from the healthy life you want to live, with **shoulder freedom**.

Here is thing, shoulder problems are **cumulative**. Meaning they take time. A series of choices made (or not made) lead to shoulder pain, and injuries. Today, we are going to stop shoulder pain. And most importantly, turn your shoulder into a durable castle of health.

First, we will discuss the **shoulder anatomy**. This will help you understand the complex structure of the shoulder. We will discuss shoulder bone structure, the joint, muscles and ligaments. The more you can appreciate intricate workings of your shoulder, the easier you can make smart decisions for future shoulder health.

Then we will move into the rotator cuff. Which holds the "gleno-humeral joint together." We will talk about the four main muscle of the rotator cuff (supraspinatus, infraspinatus, teres minor and subscapularis) and get into their function.

Next we will define different movements of the shoulder and how the rotator cuff is utilized throughout these movements. Appropriate movement definition will aid in direction for the exercises listed in this book. Then we will touch on shoulder stability, and the different types.

Then we get into specific types of injuries and what occurs when you injure your shoulder. Particularly what happens when you injure your rotator cuff. We will discuss instability, impingements, inflammation, calcium deposits and tears. Injuries happen. Our goal is avoid them. This guide will help you achieve (and maintain) shoulder strength, durability and health.

After that, we will get into dynamic warm ups and shoulder stretches. Shoulder stretches are a huge aspect to this guide because rotator cuff flexibility is a very important part of shoulder health.

Then after we talk about shoulder stretches, we get into shoulder strength training. There is a large variety of shoulder strength training moves and concepts for the rotator cuff. You will use light dumbbells (5 pounds), and resistance bands. These moves will progress from simple and low difficulty, to complex and more difficult. It is very important that you progress slowly and not rush into more advanced moves. If you are coming out of injury or pain, execute easy moves. As you gain strength, move into more advanced moves.

This guide will give you every exercise you need for a strong, durable and healthy rotator cuff. How you use these workouts, is as important as what exercises you execute. Be cautious and progress slowly. Before you know it, you will feel strong and healthy. That healthy state is when you achieve, **shoulder freedom**. I wish you the very best. -Zach

THE SHOULDER – ANATOMY

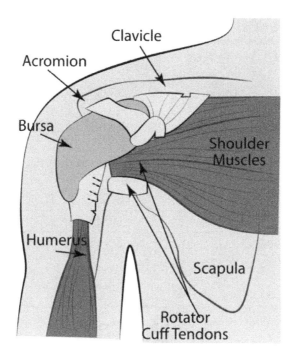

The shoulder is one of the most vital and essential body parts for conducting motions and movements. The shoulders are multi-directional and, due to their particular anatomy, they are capable of moving in all four directions – upwards, downwards, forwards and backwards – as well as being able to rotate in circular motions.

The basic anatomy of the shoulder will now be defined using illustrations for better understanding of the structure.

Shoulder Bones

Figure 1 shows the basic structure of the shoulder. There are three main bones attached at a 90-degree angle to create the shoulder joint. These are as listed below.

1. **Humerus**: the bone in the upper arm

2. **Scapula**: the shoulder blade

3. **Clavicle**: the collarbone

These bones are joined together to make two different joints. Along with each bone, there are attached muscles that provide extra protection and aid in movement.

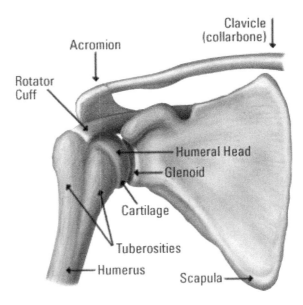

Figure 1 – Structure of the Shoulder

Shoulder Joints:

The three bones of the shoulders make two joints, which are the gleno-humeral joint and the acromio-clavicular joint. *Figure 2* shows, that the connection between the arm and the scapula (*shoulder blade*) make a gleno-humeral joint. The joint between the scapula and clavicle (*collarbone*) make the acromo-clavicular joint.

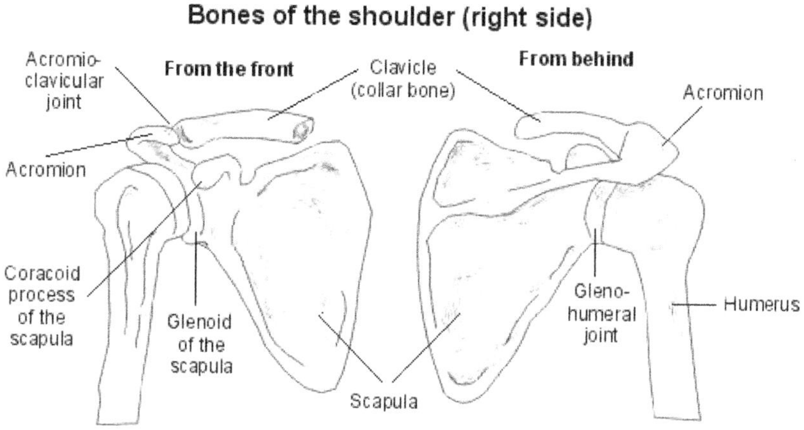

Bones of the shoulder (right side)

Figure 2 – Joint in Shoulder Muscles

Shoulder Muscles and Ligaments:

The body is composed of four main elements, which collectively create the structure of the human skeleton. These are the bones, muscles, tendons and ligaments. A **muscle** is made up of tissues that contract and relax in accordance with nerve signals. A **tendon** connects muscles with bones and a **ligament** connects bones with bones.

Many muscles hold the shoulder joint together. The most important of all is the rotator muscle and the acromio-clavicular ligaments, as well as the gleno-humeral joint capsule – as shown in *Figure 3*. The gleno-humeral joint capsule is a ball and socket joint that is formed by the humerus and scapula. This joint helps in the circular rotation of the arm, as well as its upward and downward movement. It also allows the arm to move freely in the socket.

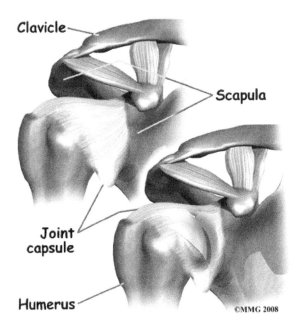

Clavicle

Scapula

Joint
capsule

Humerus

©MMG 2008

Figure 3 – Gleno-humeral Joint Capsule

The other surrounding muscles in the area also support the movement of the shoulder. They are the deltoid shoulder muscle, pectoralis major (chest muscles), teres major, lattissimus dorsi, biceps and triceps. The biceps allow the elbow to bend instantly while the other six muscles help with rotator cuff injuries and conditions. The deltoid muscles constitute of the anterior fiber, posterior fiber and middle fiber. The deltoid anterior fiber flexes the shoulder and horizontally abducts it. The posterior fiber deltoid helps in the extension of the muscle and abducts the shoulder horizontally. Finally, the middle deltoid fiber abducts the shoulder.

The Rotator Cuff

The rotator cuff is a set of muscles and tendons that hold the gleno-humeral joint together. This group helps the movement of the arm in all directions. *Figure 4* illustrates the location of the muscles.

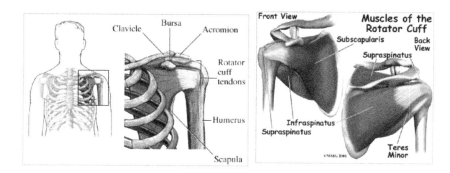

Figure 4 – The Rotator Cuff

A rotator muscle (*Figure 5*) comprises of four major muscles, namely the supraspinatus, infraspinatus, teres minor and subscapularis. They stabilize the shoulder; if any of the four do not perform their function, then shoulder movement becomes impossible.

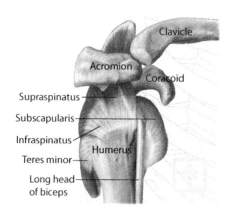

Figure 5 – Four Major Rotation Cuff Muscles

ROTATOR CUFF MOVEMENT

R otation cuff movement is a complex phenomenon. Each muscle helps in the movement of the shoulder in different directions. Supraspinatus muscles help the arm move in the side directions of the body. It originates above the spine of the scapula and inserts into the humerus. It also helps in the elevation of the arm.

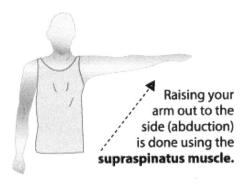

Raising your arm out to the side (abduction) is done using the **supraspinatus muscle.**

The infraspinatus and teres minor in the humerus allow external rotation. The infraspinatus originates from below the scapula spine and inserts into the posterior of the humerus. The teres minor originates from the lateral scapula board and inserts into the inferior humerus.

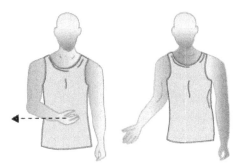

The **infraspinatus and teres minor muscle** allow you to rotate your arm and shoulder away from your body.

The subscapularis helps in the internal rotation of the arm. It originates from the anterior surface of the scapula, thus covering the ribs and inserting into the humerus.

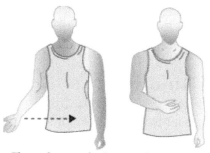

The **subscapularis muscle** is used
when the arm and shoulder rotate
towards the body.

All these muscles work together with the rotator cuff to stabilize the movement of the shoulder joint and the gleno-humeral joint.

Stabilizer – Rotator Cuff Movement

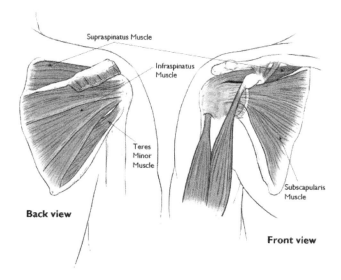

Supraspinatus Muscle

Infraspinatus Muscle

Teres Minor Muscle

Subscapularis Muscle

Back view

Front view

The stability of the shoulder is one of the most important traits of the shoulder. The shoulder is held in place by two main stabilizers: the dynamic stabilizer (muscles) and the static stabilizers (ligaments and capsule). During shoulder movement, there is a chance of overstretching the static stabilizers. To avoid such damage, there should appropriate care applied when stretching your shoulder.

Rotator Cuff Injuries

Normal rotator cuff pain is observed in all kinds of people, regardless of age. The pain may be acute or minor, and may even result in serious injuries like tendon tearing. Advanced studies and techniques are being used to identify the cause of this damage. Also many people are working hard to reduce the inefficiency of the shoulder treatment.

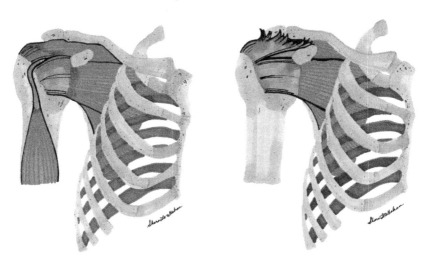

Normal Rotation Cuff   **Rotation Cuff Tear**

Normal tearing in the shoulder rotation cuff is illustrated above.

Many exercises and stretches can help promote a quick recovery of rotator cuff muscles (which we will get to in this book). There is specific exercises and stretches that can increase your speed of recovery and increase your shoulder durability. Without proper care, here are some injuries that can occur.

COMMON SHOULDER INJURIES

The shoulder comprises of different bones, muscles, tendons and ligaments. The movement of the shoulder can be hindered if there is any injury in these components. These injuries are more common in athletes or people who exercise excessively (especially overhead throwing athletes). Such injuries can result in acute pain and hindrance in joint movement; injuries can become complicated and complex if not treated in time.

Normal rotation cuff pain is observed in all people of different ages. This could be acute or minor pain, or result in serious injury like tears to the tendons, which can hinder the full rotation of the shoulder (Always consult a medical professional when you experience pain). Many studies and techniques are used to identify and treat the cause in order to reduce the inefficiency of the shoulder.

Impingement in the shoulder rotation cuff is illustrated below.

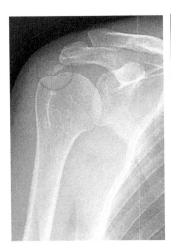 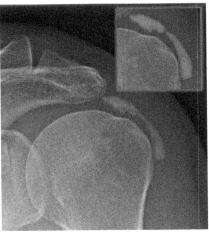

Some commonly observed injuries are as follows:

Injury Types

Instability

Shoulder instability occurs when the shoulder is moved from its original position, which is a condition that can result in dislocation of any joint in the muscles. People who are suffering from shoulder instability will feel pain in their shoulder joint during any shoulder-related movement. In worse conditions, a person may also feel that the shoulder joint is slipping from its place. This causes instability in the arm and results in lesser movement and flexibility of the joints. Repetitive strain is the result of increased loosening of ligaments in the shoulder muscles. Swimming, tennis and volleyball are the sports that require continuous overhead movement that can stretch the shoulder ligaments. Some jobs also involve repetitive overhead work. There is also multidirectional instability in some patients; their joints may be dislocated from the front, back or sides.

Impingement

Due to excessive overhead arm movement, the shoulder muscles may frequently rub with the upper part of shoulder blade (*acromion*) and cause impingement. There are several reasons why impingement occurs, including muscle weakness, individual anatomy and the angle of muscle movement. Muscle weakness is the result of not pulling the head of humerus sufficiently enough to raise the arm. There are differences in all people and their respective structures. Some people have less space between their humerus and acromion, which results in lesser movement in arm or shoulder rotation. There are many examples where these problems can be faced, such as during swimming or throwing. All these activities involve the external and internal rotation of the shoulder muscles.

Because of impingement, there may be lesser space for the arm to complete internal or external movement.

Inflammation

Due to excessive exercise or shoulder stress, the soft shoulder muscles may become inflamed. There are different types of inflammation, such as bursitis, which is a soft sac-like structure that cushions between the ball of the humerus and the socket of the G-H joint. Inflammation in any of the rotator cuff tendons is called tendonitis. The covering of bone (*perisosteum*) is called periostitis.

Calcium deposits

This is the condition in which calcium is deposited in the muscle or tendon. The accumulation of calcium can result in stress and muscle inflammation. When calcium begins accumulating in the shoulder, it forms special types of "-its", which are responsible for inflammation in soft muscles. This condition takes the form of muscles tears.

Tears

Ligament tearing is known as a sprain while muscle tearing is known as a strain. A tear that pulls a tendon off the bone at its insertion site is called an avulsion. When dealing with muscle tearing, there is intense shoulder pain. The tearing could be a result of heavy lifting or falling. When the injury occurs, muscle spasms take place; these are a bodily response referred to as "guarding" or "splinting". This guarding of the muscles helps the body to avoid extending the arm by more than 45 degrees; if this were to happen, you would feel a very strong sensation of pain that would hinder their shoulder muscle movement. If there is acute tearing in the shoulder muscles, surgical treatment may be administered. The two major types of tears that are observed in people are partial tears and full-thickness tears. The former is a slight tear in the soft tissue while the second involves the muscles breaking into two pieces

Arthritis

Shoulder pain can also be the result of arthritis. The most common type of arthritis in the shoulders is called osteoarthritis, which is also known as "wear and tear" arthritis. The early symptoms are shoulder pain, stiffness and swelling. Osteoarthritis develops over time and is usually diagnosed during middle age.

Fracture

In younger patients, a shoulder fracture is usually the result of a fall or severe injuries.

GETTING STARTED: WARM-UP

Warm-up

Before starting any kind of exercise, warm up your body. Just 10 to 15 minutes of simple walking, cycling or running can warm up the shoulders and chest muscles. This warm-up helps blood to begin circulating gently around your body.

It is necessary to do this before any workout because it prevents injuries to the muscles, tendons and ligaments. A perfect warm-up will increase the blood and body temperature, which results in faster muscle response.

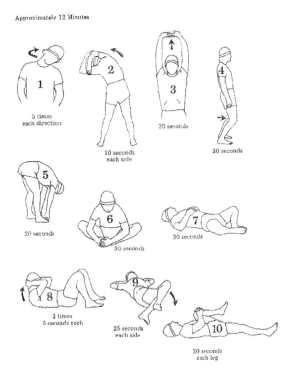

Approximately 12 Minutes

1
5 times
each direction

2
10 seconds
each side

3
20 seconds

4
30 seconds

5
20 seconds

6
30 seconds

7
30 seconds

8
3 times
5 seconds each

9
25 seconds
each side

10
20 seconds
each leg

The above figures show some simple exercises to help you warm up your body before following up with rotator cuff exercises.

You have freedom to choose how you warm up your body. The most important part, start to break a sweat!

SHOULDER STRETCHES

The first section of rotator cuff exercises is focused on stretching the shoulder. You will particularly notice many static stretches. Static stretches are meant to be held with a certain amount of force. It is important to hold static stretches for at least 10 full seconds.

You do not have to start with static stretches. But I prefer starting off my exercise routine with my favorite static stretches. This way I am promoting much needed flexibility.

Flexibility is one of the main drivers for rotator cuff health. Strength workouts are also very important. But we will discuss those later in this book.

Do no neglect shoulder flexibility. The more you stretch, the more flexibility and mobility you will achieve. This will promote long term shoulder health.

Shoulder Rotating Forward - Arms to the Side

Instructions: Place your arms at your side and relax your shoulder muscles. Stand in an upright position. Begin moving your shoulders in a circular motion. First, lift your shoulders up and then move them forwards. Finally, relax back into the original position. Repeat this process for a total of 10 reps.

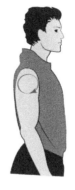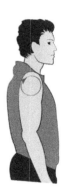

Focus: Your focus should be on rotating your shoulders in a forward motion.

Feeling: Make big circular motions so that it stretches the back and chest muscles, thus resulting in the uplift of the body. For better results, relax the muscles, which are directly involved in the movement. This allows the muscles to stretch easily without any stiffness and also allows your body to relax. With this exercise, you will feel rotation and movement in the clavicle.

Key points: Take your time during this exercise, but keep your back straight and firm. Breath in and out deeply while you perform an action.

Time or Reps: Make 10 circular rounds in the same direction at a continuous pace.

Difficulty level: 1 of 5

Shoulder Rotating Backward – Arms to the Side

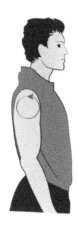 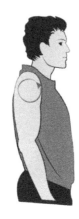

Instructions: Stand tall with a straight back, lift both shoulders and rotate your shoulders backwards in a large and smooth circular motion. Involve your chest muscles to uplift the upper body and relax your back muscles when moving in a backward motion.

Focus: Your focus should be on rotating your shoulders in backward rotating motion.

Feeling: Make big circular motions, so that the back and chest muscles are stretched to achieve an uplift of the body. For better results, relax the muscles that are directly involved in the movement. This will allow the muscles to stretch without any stiffness, thus allowing your body to relax. With this exercise, you will feel rotation and movement in the clavicle.

Key points: Take your time, but keep your back straight and firm. Take a deep breath in and out while you perform each action. During exercise, inhale from the nose and exhale from the mouth.

Time or Reps: Make 10 circular rounds in the same direction at a continuous pace.

Difficulty level: 1 of 5

Neck Rotation to the Right

Instructions: To stretch your neck muscles, stand straight and then gently bend your neck towards your chest. As you do this, relax your body and then gently move your neck to the right side. Bring back your position back to the similar posture of dropping your neck towards your chest, and then repeat the process. Keep your neck muscles relaxed and do not stiffen your neck. Keep your neck in the right direction and stretch it gently.

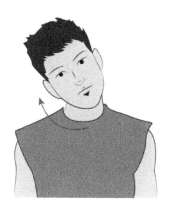

Focus: Your focus should be on keeping your neck in the right direction without bending it.

Feeling: You should feel your neck stretching along with the trapezius muscles.

Key points: Do not throw back your head roughly or you might strain your neck.

During the exercise, inhale from the nose and exhale from the mouth.

Time or Reps: Move your neck 5 times in a similar direction.

Difficulty Level: 1 of 5

Neck Rotation to the Left

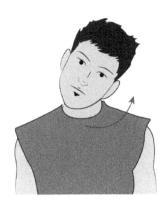

Instructions: To stretch your neck muscles, stand straight and gently bend your neck towards your chest. At the same time, relax your body and gently move your neck to the left side. Bring back your position to the similar posture of dropping your neck towards your chest, and then repeat the process. Keep your neck muscles relaxed and do not stiffen your neck. Keep your neck in the right direction and stretch it gently to relax the neck muscles. During the exercise, inhale from the nose and exhale from the mouth.

Focus: Your focus should be on keeping the neck in the right direction without bending it.

Feeling: You should feel your neck stretching with the trapezius muscles.

Key points: Do not throw back your head in a manner that might strain it. During the exercise, inhale from the nose and exhale from the mouth.

Time or Reps: Move your neck 5 times in a similar direction.

Difficulty level: 1 of 5

Arm Extension Up and Hold

Instructions: Stand straight and keep your feet shoulder width apart. Bring both arms over your head and hold your hands. Stretch your arms upwards and hold this position for 10 to 15 seconds.

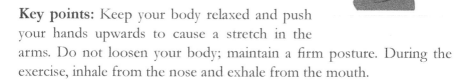

Focus: Your focus should be on holding your arms straight and firm.

Feeling: You will feel stretching in your shoulder, lats and forearms.

Key points: Keep your body relaxed and push your hands upwards to cause a stretch in the arms. Do not loosen your body; maintain a firm posture. During the exercise, inhale from the nose and exhale from the mouth.

Time or Reps: Hold for 10 seconds and keep your breathing constant.

Difficulty level: 1 of 5

Arm Circles Forward - Small

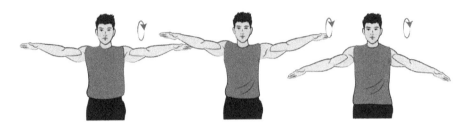

Instructions: Stand straight and hold your arms level with your shoulders. Make a 90-degree angle to the floor. This is the starting positing for your exercise. Now slowly make small circles with both arms in forward-pointing position.

When making smaller circles with your arms, the neck and back shoulders are in a constant circular motion.

Focus: You should focus on keeping your body straight and make a complete small circular motion.

Feeling: You will feel pressure in the biceps and triceps and the full movement of the rotator cuff. The movement of all four muscles should give stability and support to the shoulder joint. You will feel a slight burning sensations in your rotator cuff.

Key points: Maintain a proper posture and stretch your arms completely in a 90-degree angle. Keep a constant pace while making smaller circles. Keep your breathing normal and take your time to easily complete one rotation. With a circle that is smaller in diameter, there will be less tension between the arm function and rotation. This version of exercise is used to loosen the arm and shoulder muscles. During this exercise, inhale from the nose and exhale from the mouth.

Time or Reps: Repeat this process 10 times, making circular motions in a forward direction.

Difficulty level: 1 of 5

Arm Circles Backward - Small

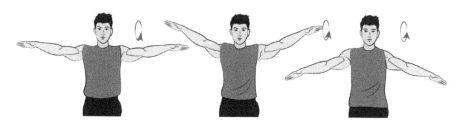

Instructions: Stand straight and hold your arms at the same level as your shoulders. Make a 90-degree angle to the floor; this is the starting positing for your exercise. Now, slowly make small circles with both arms in a backward position. When making smaller circles with your arms, the neck and back shoulders are in a constant circular motion.

Focus: You should focus on keeping your body straight and on making a complete circular motion backwards.

Feeling: You will feel pressure in the biceps and triceps and the full movement of the rotation cuff. The movement of all the four muscles would give stability and support to the shoulder joint. You will feel a slight burning sensations in your rotator cuff.

Key points: Maintain a proper posture and stretch your arms completely in a 90-degree angle. Keep a constant pace while making smaller circles and maintain your breathing at a normal pace, while taking your time to complete one rotation.

With a smaller circle, there is less tension created between the arm function and rotation. This version of exercise is used to loosen the muscles in the arms and shoulders. During this exercise, inhale from the nose and exhale from the mouth. You can increase speed as your shoulder loosens.

Time or Reps: Repeat this process 10 times, making circular motions in a backward direction.

Difficulty level: 1 of 5

Arm Circles Forward - Big

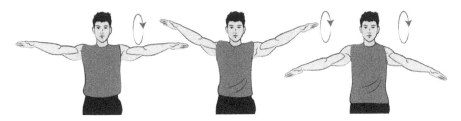

Instructions: Stand straight and hold your arms on the same level as your shoulders. Make a 90-degree angle to the floor; this is the starting positing for your exercise. Slowly make larger circles with both arms in a forward position. When making larger circles, your arms, neck and back shoulders are in constant motion providing dynamic stretching and loosening to the shoulder muscles.

Focus: You should focus on keeping your body straight and on making a complete circular motion.

Feeling: You will feel pressure in the biceps and triceps and the full movement of the rotation cuff. The movement of all four muscles will give stability and support to the shoulder joint. Inward and outward movement of the shoulder muscles cause a dynamic stretch in the entire joint.

Key points: Maintain a proper posture and stretch your arms completely in a 90-degree angle. Keep a constant pace while making larger circles. Keep your breathing normal at this point and take your time to easily complete one rotation. During a larger circle, there is more tension created between the arm function and rotation. This version of exercise pumps blood into the muscles of your arms and shoulders. During the exercise, inhale from the nose and exhale from the mouth.

Time or Reps: Repeat this process 10 times, making circular motion in a forward direction.

Difficulty level: 1 of 5

Arm Circles Backward - Big

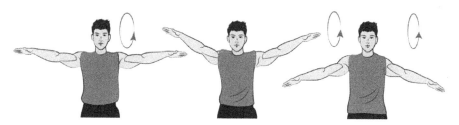

Instructions: Stand straight and hold your arms level to your shoulders. Make a 90-degree angle to the floor as the starting positing for the exercise. Take your palms and turn them skyward. Now make larger circles with both arms in a backward position. When making larger circles, your arms, neck and back shoulders are in a constant motion. This provides dynamic stretching and loosening of the shoulder. Especially the front of the shoulder.

Focus: You should focus on keeping your arms straight and make a complete circular motion. You may increase speed as you feel comfortable.

Feeling: You will feel pressure in the biceps and triceps and the full movement of the rotator cuff. The movement of all four muscles will give stability and support to the shoulder joint. Inward and outward movement of the shoulder muscles should cause a dynamic stretch to the entire joint.

Key points: Maintain a proper posture and stretch your arms completely in a 90-degree angle. Keep a constant pace while making larger circles. Keep your breathing normal at this point and take your time to easily complete one rotation. At a larger circle, there is more tension created between the arm function and rotation. This version of exercise pumps blood to the muscles in the arms and shoulders. During the exercise, inhale from the nose and exhale from the mouth.

Time or Reps: Repeat this process 10 times, making circular motion in a backward direction.

Difficulty level: 1 of 5

Right Arm Across and Hold

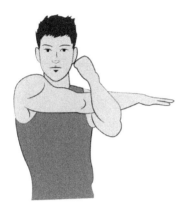

Instructions: Keep your back and posture straight with your feet shoulder width apart. Bring your right arm close to your chest and lift your left hand. Pull your arm towards your chest and hold. Keep your shoulders straight while you stretch your arm. Feel the stretch across your deltoid and deep in your rotator cuff. As you press your arm against your chest inhale from your nose and exhale through your mouth.

Focus: You should focus on pulling your arm towards your chest. An extra clinch of the bicep can make a big difference

Feeling: You should feel deep stretch in the deltoid and rotator cuff of the shoulder

Key points: Keep your body in an upright position. Do not reduce the pressure across the arm. Stretch to your comfort zone. During the exercise, inhale from the nose and exhale from the mouth.

Time or reps: Count 10 to 20 seconds and then release.

Difficulty level: 1 of 5

Left Arm Across and Hold

Instructions: Keep your back and posture straight with your feet shoulder width apart. Bring your left arm up close to your chest and lift your right hand. Pull your arm towards your chest and hold. Keep your shoulders straight while you stretch your arm. Feel the stretch across your deltoid and deep in your rotator cuff. As you press your arm against your chest inhale from your nose and exhale through your mouth.

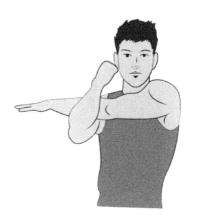

Focus: You should focus on pulling your arm towards your chest. An extra clinch of the bicep can make a big difference

Feeling: You should feel deep stretch in the deltoid and rotator cuff of the shoulder

Key points: Keep your body in an upright position. Do not reduce the pressure across the arm. Stretch to your comfort zone. During the exercise, inhale from the nose and exhale from the mouth.

Time or reps: Count 10 to 20 seconds and then release.

Difficulty level: 1 of 5

Right Arm Overhead and Hold

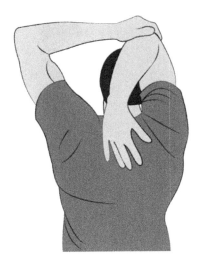

Instructions: Stand straight with good posture. Keep your feet shoulder width apart. Straighten your back and lift your right hand over your head. Bend your arm at the elbow joint and hold the elbow with the left hand. Place your right hand's fingers on the shoulder blade area. Feel the stretch in your right triceps and keep your shoulders loose.

Focus: You should focus on pulling your elbow straight back behind your head. Keep it in place with the left hand. Reach your fingers down the back of your shoulder blades.

Feeling: You should feel deep stretch on your lats, triceps and rotator cuff.

Key points: Keep your posture up. Flex your right bicep to add an extra stretch.

Keep your breathing constant. Inhale from your nose and exhale from your mouth.

Difficulty Level: 2 of 5

Left Arm Overhead and Hold

Instructions: Stand straight with good posture. Keep your feet shoulder width apart. Straighten your back and lift your left hand over your head. Bend your arm at the elbow joint and hold the elbow with the right hand. Place your left hand's fingers on the shoulder blade area. Feel the stretch in your left triceps and lat. Keep your shoulders loose.

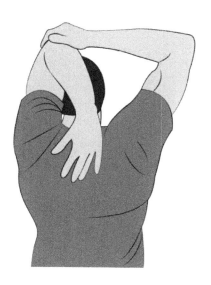

Focus: You should focus on pulling your elbow straight back behind your head. Keep it in place with the right hand. Reach your fingers down the back of your shoulder blades.

Feeling: You should feel deep stretch on your lats, triceps and rotator cuff.

Key points: Keep your posture up. Flex your left bicep to add an extra stretch.

Keep your breathing constant. Inhale from your nose and exhale from your mouth.

Time or Reps: Count 10 seconds and release. Stretch to your comfort zone.

Difficulty Level: 2 of 5

Right Arm Across by Opposite Hip and Hold

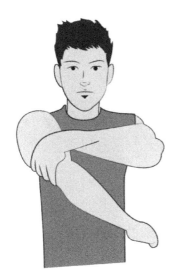

Instructions: Stand in a firm upright position. Keep your feet apart. Hold your right arm across the opposite hip and hold from the left hand at the elbow of your right hand.

Focus: Your focus should be pulling your arm down by the opposite hip. You can move your neck and feel a deeper stretch.

Feeling: You should feel a deep stretch on your posterior cuff, traps and scapula.

Key points: Keep your shoulders firm during the stretch. Move your neck for a deeper stretch.

Time and Reps: Count 10 seconds and drop your hand.

Difficulty level: 1 of 5

Left Arm Across Opposite Hip and Hold

Instructions: Stand in a firm position and keeping your feet apart. Pull your left arm across your chest toward your opposite hip. Hold your arm on the opposite hip and support your left arm by holding it from the elbow with your right hand.

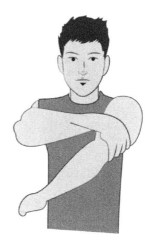

Focus: Your focus should be on holding your arm firmly at its place. Stretch your left arm to the opposite hip.

Feeling: You will feel a deep stretch to the biceps, triceps and scapula.

Key points: Keep your shoulders firm during the workout and inhale from the nose and exhale from the mouth. Stretch to your comfort zone. Move neck down towards opposite hip to feel a deep stretch.

Time and Reps: Count 10 seconds and then release.

Difficulty level: 1 of 5

Right Arm Extension Stretch

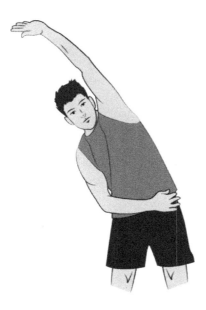

Instructions: Stand straight with your feet shoulder width apart. Lean down to your left side and kick out your opposite hip. Bring your right arm over your head. Stretch it outwards and keep your posture aligned straight. Stretch yourself upwards to the left.

Focus: Your focus should be on keeping your are extended without bending into an arch shape.

Feeling: You should feel a tight stretch all the way from your shoulders to your arms, ribcage and lat.

Key points: You should bend to the left side. Keep your hips kicked outwards on the right side. Keep calm and hold the position. Inhale and exhale smoothly while holding.

Time or Reps: Keep this position, count 10 seconds and then release your position.

Difficulty level: 2 of 5

Left Arm Extension Stretch

Instructions: Stand straight with your feet shoulder width apart. Lean down to your right side and kick out your opposite hip. Bring your left arm over your head. Stretch it outwards and keep your posture aligned straight. Stretch yourself upwards to the right.

Focus: Your focus should be on keeping your are extended without bending into an arch shape.

Feeling: You should feel a tight stretch all the way from your shoulders to your arms, ribcage and lat.

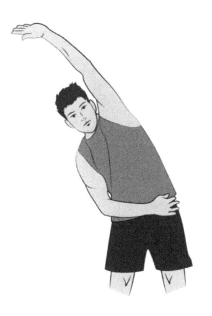

Key points: You should bend to the right side. Keep your hips kicked outwards on the left side. Keep calm and hold the position. Inhale and exhale smoothly while holding.

Time or Reps: Keep this position, count 10 seconds and then release your position.

Difficulty level: 2 of 5

Sleeper Stretch – Right Arm

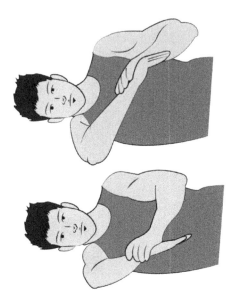

Instructions: Lie down on your right side, bend your knees. Bend your right arm. Your elbow should be facing the shoulder at 90-degree angle. Using your left hand, press down your right arm.

Focus: Your focus should be on keeping your elbow bent at 90 degrees. While pressing down on your hand. Your arm should not bend inwards; it should remain at a 90 degree angle. The pressure on your arm should be gentle.

Feeling: You should feel a deep stretch in the shoulder, back and shoulder capsule.

Key points: Press down on the right arm behind the wrist. Do not push too hard. Be careful with this stretch. Keep your breathing normal.

Time and Reps: Hold this position for 10 seconds and release.

Difficulty level: 2 of 5

Sleeper Stretch - Left Arm

Instructions: Lie down on your left side, bend your knees. Bend your left arm. Your elbow should be facing the shoulder at 90-degree angle. Using your right hand, press down your left arm.

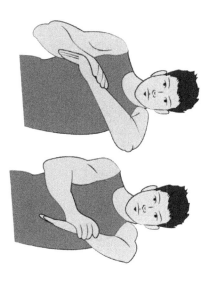

Focus: Your focus should be on keeping your elbow bent at 90 degrees. While pressing down on your hand. Your arm should not bend inwards; it should remain at a 90 degree angle. The pressure on your arm should be gentle.

Feeling: You should feel a deep stretch in the shoulder, back and shoulder capsule.

Key points: Press down on the left arm behind the wrist. Do not push too hard. Be careful with this stretch. Keep your breathing normal.

Time and Reps: Hold this position for 10 seconds and release. Make 3 reps.

Difficulty level: 2 of 5

Lat Pull Stretch - Right Arm

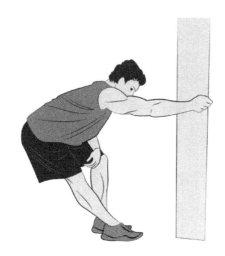

Instructions: Find a pole that you can grip firmly. Hold the pole with your right hand, bend your neck and lean backwards using your body weight. Lean back to your full arm length. Place your left hand on your left leg. Stretching your right leg, use your hips to pull yourself backwards. Use your legs to maintain your balance by keeping your feet together. Now use your body weight to pull backwards.

Focus: Your focus should be on keeping your right arm straight and using your body weight to stretch. Push your body backwards while holding the pole.

Feeling: You should feel your lat muscles stretching, along with your rotator cuff and all the muscles located at the back of your shoulder.

Key points: Keep your back straight maintain good posture. Use your hips to pull your body back into the right position. Keep your breathing constant.

Time or Reps: Hold this position for 10 seconds.

Difficulty level: 2 of 5

Lat Pull Stretch - Left Arm

Instructions: Find a pole that you can grip on firmly. Hold the pole with your left hand, bend your neck and lean backwards with the help of your body weight. Place your right hand on your right leg. Stretch your left leg using your hips to push backwards. Use your legs to maintain your balance by keeping your feet together.

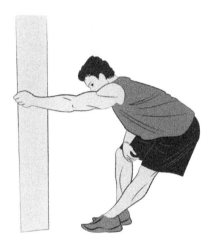

Now start using your body weight to pull backwards with your left elbow moving towards your left hip.

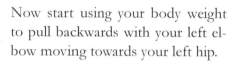

Focus: Your focus should be on keeping your left arm straight and using your body weight to stretch. Push your body backwards while holding the pole.

Feeling: You should feel your lat muscles stretching, along with your rotator cuff and all the muscles located at the back of your shoulder. This also stretches your shoulder blade area.

Key points: Keep your back straight. Use your hips to push back your body in the right position. Keep your breathing constant.

Time or Reps: Hold this position for 10 seconds.

Difficulty level: 2 of 5

Lat Extensions With Exercise Ball

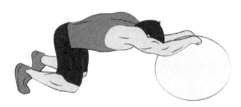

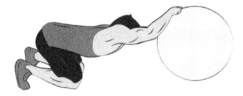

Instructions: Sit on your knees and place your arms on a physio ball. Roll out until your back is straight. Stretch your arms to their complete length. Apply pressure on the ball.

Focus: You should focus on keeping pressure on your arms and on the floor with the help of your knees.

Feeling: You should feel pressure building in your lat muscles and the shoulder muscles behind your back.

Key points: You can roll the ball on your sides with your hands. While applying the pressure on the ball with your hands, stretch your body backwards.

Time or Reps: Take 10 to 15 seconds during one rep. Complete 3 reps.

Difficulty level: 3 of 5

Lat Extension With Foam Roller

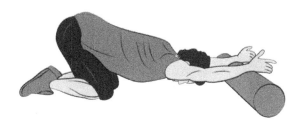

Instructions: Sit on your knees and place your arms on the foam roller. Roll out until your back is straight. Stretch your arms to their complete length. Apply pressure on the foam roller.

Focus: You should focus on keeping pressure on your arms on the floor with the help of your knees.

Feeling: You should feel pressure building in your lat muscles and the shoulder muscles behind your back.

Key points: You can roll the foam roller front and back using your hands. While applying the pressure on the foam roller with your hands, stretch your body backwards and forwards.

Time or Reps: Take 10 to 15 seconds during one rep. Complete 3 reps.

Difficulty level: 2 of 5

Foam Roll Over Lat Massage - Right Arm

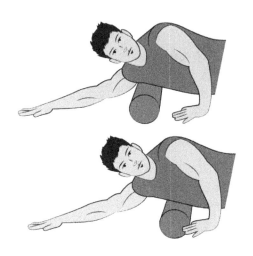

Instructions: Lay on your side and place the foam under your arm pit on the lat muscle. Stretch your arm and lift your body over the foam with your other hand on the floor in front of your chest. Use your hand to lean on the ground and support your upper body. Using your legs, slowly move forwards and backwards. This will allow a smoother massage for your lat.

Focus: Your focus should be on placing your body at a right angle and maintaining the pressure on the foam roller with your upper body.

Feeling: You should feel pressure on your lat muscle behind your shoulder. This will loosen the lat area.

Key points: Your arms and legs will help you to support your body pressure onto the roller.

Time or Reps: Continue this workout for 10-15 seconds and resume your position. Complete 2 to 3 reps.

Difficulty level: 3 of 5

Foam Roll Over Lat Massage - Left Arm

Instructions: Lay on your side place the foam roller under your left armpit. Stretch your arm and lift your body over the foam with your other hand in front of your chest. Use your hand to lean on the ground and support your upper body. Using your legs, slowly move forwards and backwards. This will allow a smoother massage to your upper lat.

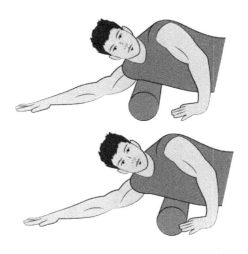

Focus: Your focus should be on placing your body at a right angle and maintaining the pressure on the foam with your upper body.

Feeling: You should feel pressure on your lat muscle behind your shoulder. This will loosen the lat area.

Key points: Your arms and legs will help you to support your body pressure.

Time or Reps: Continue rolling for 10-15 seconds.

Complete 2 to 3 reps.

Difficulty level: 3 of 5

Shoulders Back

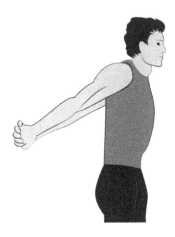

Instructions: Stand straight, keep your feet together, relax your body and straighten your shoulders. Pull back your arms at a 30-degree angle. Stretch your arms back and hold the position.

Focus: Your focus should be on keeping your back straight, widening your chest and stretching your arms straight in a backwards direction.

Feeling: You should feel pressure on your shoulder blades. Your biceps and triceps should be stretching as you push your arms behind your back. Your clavicle will also stretch and your ribcage will lift upwards.

Key points: Keep pressure at a comfort zone. Bigger muscles may hinder flexibility here. Inhale and exhale in smooth manner.

Time or Reps: Continue this workout for 10-15 seconds and then release.

Difficulty level: 2 of 5

Posterior Cuff Stretch – Left Arm

Instructions: Stand straight and put your left arm behind your lower back with the elbow pointing outwards. Keep your back straight. With your right hand, hold the elbow of your left arm and gently pull it forwards.

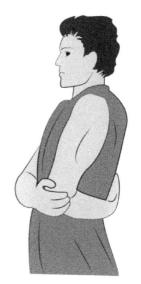

Focus: Your focus should be on keeping your back straight and keeping your arm steady behind your lower back.

Feeling: You should feel stretching in your posterior cuff.

Key points: Keep your back and shoulders straight. Stretch to your comfort zone. Move your hand up or down your back based on your tolerance. Be very easy with this stretch.

Time or Reps: Keep this workout for 5 - 10 seconds and then resume your position.

Difficulty level: 2 of 5

Posterior Cuff Stretch – Right Arm

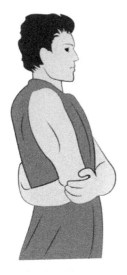

Instructions: Stand straight and put your right arm behind your lower back with the elbow pointing outwards. Keep your back straight. With your left hand, hold the elbow of your left arm and gently pull it forwards.

Focus: Your focus should be on keeping your back straight and keeping your arm steady behind your lower back.

Feeling: You should feel stretching in your posterior cuff.

Key points: Keep your back and shoulders straight. Stretch to your comfort zone. Move your hand up or down your back based on your tolerance. Be very easy with this stretch.

Time or Reps: Continue this workout for 10-15 seconds and then resume your position. Make 3 reps.

Difficulty level: 2 of 5

Chest Stretch Straight – Right Arm

Instructions: Stand straight next to a wall and place your right hand on that wall shoulder level. Now, start turning your body away from the wall until you can feel the stretch.

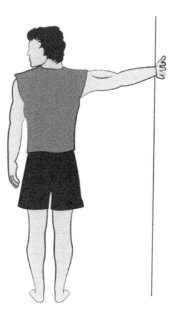

Focus: Your focus should be lengthening your chest.

Feeling: There will be a strong stretch across your chest.

Key points: Stand straight and try to practice this exercise at three different angles: above the shoulder, leveled to shoulder and below the shoulder. Stretch to your comfort zone.

Time or Reps: Hold this workout for 10-15 seconds and then release.

Difficulty level: 1 of 5

Chest Stretch Straight – Left Arm

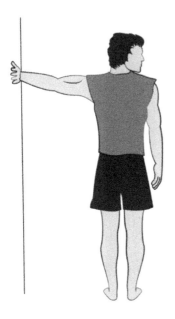

Instructions: Stand straight next to a wall and place your left arm on it, at your shoulder level. Now, start turning your body away from the wall until you feel the stretch.

Focus: Your focus should be lengthening your chest.

Feeling: There will be a strong stretch across your chest.

Key points: Stand straight and try to practice it at three different angles: above the shoulder, leveled to shoulder and below the shoulder.

Time or Reps: Continue this workout for 10-15 seconds and then release

Difficulty level: 1 of 5

Chest Stretch Elbow Bent – Right Arm

Instructions: Stand straight next to a wall and bend your right elbow at 90 degrees. At your shoulder level, place your elbow on the wall. Now, start turning your body away from the wall until you feel the stretch.

Focus: Keep your body straight while resting your arm on the wall. The arm should be firmly kept at a 90-degree angle.

Feeling: Stretch the chest and shoulder.

Key points: Keep your back straight and relax you chest. Stretch to your comfort zone.

Time or Reps: Hold this workout for 10-15 seconds and then release.

Difficulty level: 2 of 5

Chest Stretch Elbow Bent – Left Arm

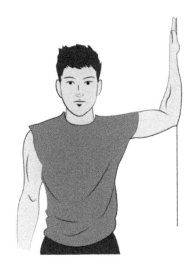

Instructions: Stand straight next to a wall and bend your left elbow at 90 degrees. At your shoulder level, place your elbow on the wall. Now, start turning your body away from the wall until you feel the stretch.

Focus: Keep your body straight and rest your arm on the wall. Your arm should be kept firmly at a 90-degree angle.

Feeling: Stretch the chest and shoulder.

Key points: Keep your back straight and relax you chest. Stretch to your comfort zone.

Time or Reps: Hold this workout for 10-15 seconds and then release.

Difficulty level: 2 of 5

Chest Stretch Arm Swing – 5 Reps

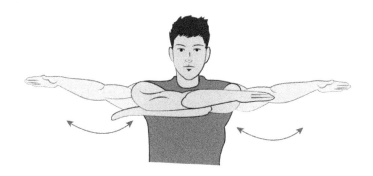

Instructions: Stand straight and cross your arms in front of your chest. Start moving both arms front and back across your body.

Focus: Your focus should be on dynamically moving your arms across your body.

Feeling: You should feel movement in both shoulders. This will loosen both arms at once.

Key points: Keep your back straight. Keep shoulders relaxed and strong. Keep your breathing normal.

Time or Reps: Keep this workout for 10-15 seconds and then resume your position. Make 5 reps.

Difficulty level: 1 of 5

Left Trap and Neck Stretch

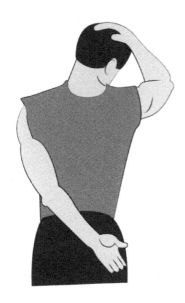

Instructions: Stand straight and place your left arm behind your back over the opposite hip. Now place your right hand over your head and bend your neck with the help of your hand.

Focus: You should focus on looking down at your right foot. Pull this slowly and feel it deep in your neck.

Feeling: You should feel stretching on your neck and trap.

Key points: Keep your back straight. Do not bend your neck in the wrong direction. Keep breathing normally. Stretch to your comfort zone.

Time or Reps: Hold this workout for 10-15 seconds and then resume your position.

Difficulty level: 2 of 5

Right Trap and Neck Stretch

Instructions: Stand straight and place your right arm behind your back over the opposite hip. Now place your left hand over your head and bend your neck with the help of your hand.

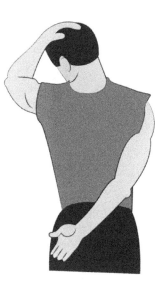

Focus: You should focus on looking down at your left foot. Pull this slowly and feel it deep in your neck.

Feeling: You should feel stretching on your neck and trap.

Key points: Keep your back straight. Do not bend your neck in the wrong direction. Keep breathing normally. Stretch to your comfort zone.

Time or Reps: Hold this workout for 10-15 seconds and then resume your position.

Difficulty level: 2 of 5

Pull Up Hang

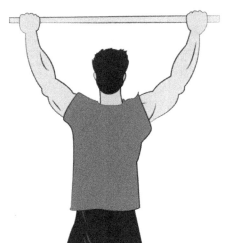

Instructions: Firmly grab hold overhead rod or pole. Set your arms apart to form a V. Now, Relax your body and feel a deep stretch in your lat.

Focus: Your arms should form a V. Have a support nearby in case this is to difficult to hold.

Feeling: Intense pressure will be felt on the lat muscles and the biceps.

Key points: Hold and breathe deep. You can vary the width of your grip.

Time or Reps: Hold for 5 to 10 seconds.

Difficulty level: 4 of 5

Lat Extension – Right Arm

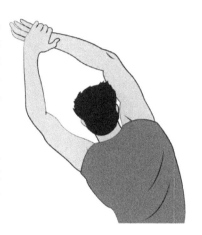

Instructions: Stand straight and lean down to your left side. Stretch your right arms over the head and hold it with your left arm. Slowly bend your body to the left side, pushing your hips in an outward direction.

Focus: Your focus should be on bending your body without forming an arch shape. Your arms should be tightly stretching their position.

Feeling: You should feel a tight stretch all the way from your shoulders, to your arms, ribcage and pelvis. Stretch to your comfort zone.

Key points: You should bend to the left side by supporting your arm with your left arm. Move your hips outwards to the right side. Keep calm and hold your position. Inhale and exhale smoothly while holding.

Time or Reps: Keep this position, count 10 seconds and then release your position.

Difficulty level: 2 of 5

Lat Extension – Left Arm

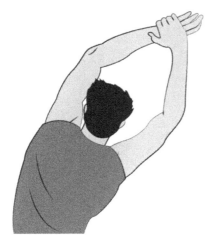

Instructions: Stand straight and lean down to your right side. Stretch your left arms over your head and hold it with your right arm. Now slowly bend your body to the right side, pushing your hips in the outward direction.

Focus: Your focus should be on bending your body without forming an arch shape. Your arms should be tightly stretching.

Feeling: You should feel a tight stretch all the way from your shoulders, to your arms, ribcage and pelvis. Stretch to your comfort zone.

Key points: You should bend to the right side by supporting your arm with the right arm. Move your hips outwards on the left side. Keep calm and hold the position. Inhale and exhale smoothly while working out.

Time or Reps: Keep this position, count 10 seconds and then release your position.

Difficulty level: 2 of 5

Towel Stretch – Right Arm

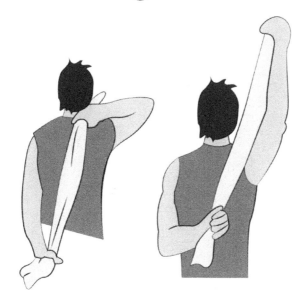

Instructions: Stand straight with your feet together. Grab a long towel and drop it over your right shoulder. Hold the shoulder in your left hand. With your right hand, hold the other end of the towel. Now gently move the towel up and down your body.

Focus: The towel should be long and your back should be straight.

Feeling: You should feel a gentle stretch on the front and the side of your shoulder. You should also feel the rotator cuff stretching.

Key points: When you feel the stretch in your shoulder, keep hold of the position and then gently leave the position.

Time or Reps: Hold this position, count 10 seconds and then release your position.

Difficulty level: 3 of 5

Towel Stretch – Left Arm

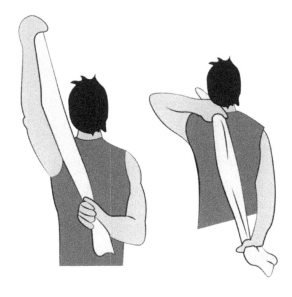

Instructions: Stand straight with your feet together. Grab a long towel and drop it over your left shoulder. Hold the towel in the right hand and hold the other end of the towel in your left hand. Now gently move the towel up and down your body.

Focus: The towel should be long and your back should be straight.

Feeling: You should feel a gentle stretch on the front and side of the shoulder. You feel the rotator cuff stretching.

Key points: When you feel the stretch in your shoulder, keep hold of the position and then gently leave the position.

Time or Reps: Hold this position for 10 seconds and then release.

Difficulty level: 3 of 5

Internal Rotation Broom Stick Stretch

Instructions: Hold a stick from one hand and position it over your head while hold the other end of the stick with the opposite arm. The arm holding the end of the stick, behind your back, should be bent from the elbow and leveled it with your shoulder.

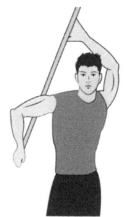

Focus: Your focus should be on holding the pole firm in its place and rotating it in an internal direction by pulling the upper end of the pole forward.

Feeling: Your will feel the stretch in the shoulder when you the pole is in a forward direction.

Key points: The elbow should be leveled to your shoulder. Maintain your breathing pattern. The forward movement of the stick would make your rotator cuff muscles more flexible.

Time or Reps: Keep this position, count 5 seconds and then release your position. Complete 3 reps.

Difficulty level: 3 of 5

RESISTANCE TRAINING - ROTATOR CUFF STRENGTH TRAINING

Now we move into my favorite part of shoulder health. **Strength training**.

Here is the rotator cuff strength mantra... **"More weight does not equal more strength."**

This means that when you focus on strengthening your rotator cuff, you only need **5 pounds** of resistance. This way you isolate your rotator cuff. Which will help you avoid using bigger muscles.

When you use a dumbbell, grab the dumbbell with your finger tips. When you use a resistance band, slower movement is always better.

The rotator cuff is going to see faster positive change based on volume of reps, not amount of weight. As you do more of the workouts, you will feel a burn in your shoulder. Especially in the posterior cuff. The burn is good. It means you are working the muscles that need to gain strength.

Be patient and develop a routine that is right for you. Some workouts are more advanced than others. Do no push yourself to hard! Know your body and you will know health.

Shoulder Flexion Thumbs Up (Right Arm)

Instructions: Stand straight with both arms straight on your side. Now hold a 5-pound weight in your right hand. Pointing your thumb up, slowly move your right arm upwards. Bring your arm to shoulder level. Hold this position for a second than slowly return to the starting position.

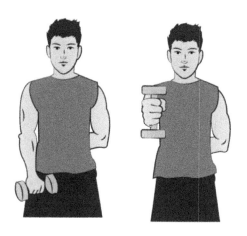

Focus: Your focus should be on keeping your arm straight and your thumb upwards.

Feeling: You should feel resistance in the front of your shoulder.

Key points: Hold the weight firmly in your hand. Breathe normally and make smooth movement upwards and downwards.

Time or Reps: Complete 3 sets of 10 reps.

Difficulty level: 1 of 5

Shoulder Flexion Thumbs Up (Left Arm)

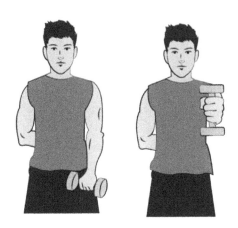

Instructions: Stand straight with both arms straight at your side. Now hold a 5-pound weight in your left hand. Pointing your thumb up, slowly move your left arm upwards. Bring your arm to your shoulder level. Hold this position for a second than slowly return to the starting position.

Focus: Your focus should be on keeping your elbow straight and your thumb upwards.

Feeling: You should feel resistance in the front of your shoulder.

Key points: Hold weight firmly in your finger tips. Breathe normally and make a smooth movement upwards and downwards.

Time or Reps: Complete 3 sets of 10 reps.

Difficulty level: 1 of 5

Shoulder Extension (Left Arm) –5 Pounds 3x10

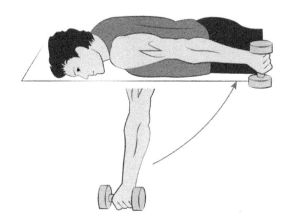

Instructions: Lean over a bench and keep your arm closer to the bench to maintain your balance. Now drop your right arm perpendicular to the floor. Hold a weight in your hand and move your arm backwards, keeping your elbow straight, towards your hips. Slowly move your arm and bring it back to the starting position.

Focus: Your focus should be on keeping your elbow straight and arm close to the body.

Feeling: You will feel resistance in your scapula, lat and posterior cuff.

Key points: Keep your elbow straight and slow movement the arm. Pinch your muscle at the top of the movement. Keep your breathing normal.

Time or Reps: Complete 3 sets of 10 reps.

Difficulty level: 2 of 5

Shoulder Extension (Right Arm) – 5 Pounds 3x10

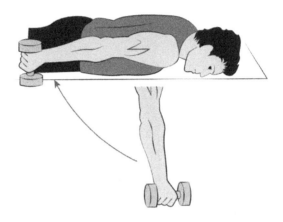

Instructions: Lean over a bench and keep your arm close to the bench. Now drop your right arm perpendicular to the floor. Hold a weight in your hand and move your arm backwards, keeping your elbow straight towards your hips. Slowly move your arm and bring it back to the starting position.

Focus: Your focus should be on keeping your elbow straight and arm closer to the body.

Feeling: You will feel resistance in your scapula, lat and posterior cuff.

Key points: Keep elbow straight and slowly move your arm. Keep your breathing normal.

Time or Reps: Complete 3 sets of 10 reps.

Difficulty level: 2 of 5

Horizontal Abduction (Right Arm) – 5 Pounds 3x10

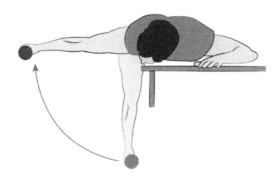

Instructions: Lean over a bench and keep your arm closer to the bench to maintain your balance. Now drop your right arm perpendicular to the floor. Hold a weight in your hand and move your arm outwards and upwards, keeping your elbow straight. Slowly move your arm and bring it back to the starting position.

Focus: Keep your elbow straight and maintain the 90 degree angle.

Feeling: You should feel resistance in your posterior cuff and scapula.

Key points: Keep your breathing normal. Move your arm away from the body you can keep your thumb up or maintain it parallel to the floor.

Time or Reps: Complete 3 sets of 10 reps.

Difficulty level: 2 of 5

Horizontal Abduction (Left Arm) – 5 Pounds 3x10

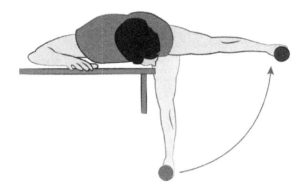

Instructions: Lean over a bench and keep your arm closer to the bench to maintain your balance. Now drop your left arm perpendicular to the floor. Hold a weight in your hand and move your arm outwards and upwards, keeping your elbow straight. Slowly move your arm and bring it back to the starting position.

Focus: Keep your elbow straight and parallel to your body.

Feeling: You should feel resistance in your posterior cuff and scapula.

Key points: Keep your breathing normal. Move your arm away from the body you can keep your thumb up or maintain it parallel to the floor.

Time or Reps: Complete 3 sets of 10 reps.

Difficulty level: 2 of 5

Shoulder Abduction – 5 Pounds 3X10

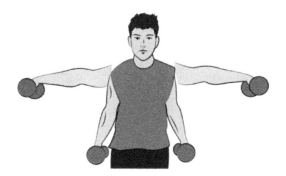

Instructions: Stand straight and keep your feet apart. Hold a weight in both hands and raise your hands parallel to the ground. Move both arms together in an upward motion. Slowly return to your starting position and repeat.

Focus: Keep your arms straight and at shoulder length when your lift your hands.

Feeling: You should feel this in the rotator cuff. The more you control the weight, the more you can feel a deep burn.

Key points: Lift your arms at your shoulder length.

Time or Reps: Complete 3 sets of 10 reps.

Difficulty level: 2 of 5

Scaption (Right Arm) – 5-Pound 3x10

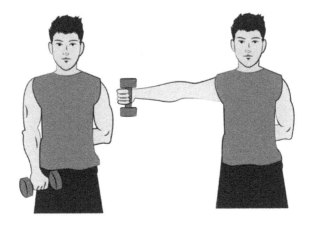

Instructions: Stand straight and keep your right arm extended and thumb up. Start raising your arm, holding weights at a 30-degree angle with your thumbs up. Bring the weight up to shoulder height Hold the position for a second then slowly return to the starting position.

Focus: Focus of the 30 degree angle in front of your body. Move slowly.

Feeling: You will feel this in the front part of your rotator cuff

Key points: Keep your balance while holding the weight. Hold the weight in your finger tips.

Time or Reps: Complete 3 sets of 10 reps.

Difficulty level: 1 of 5

Scaption (Left Arm) – 5-Pound 3x10

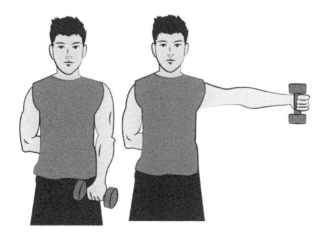

Instructions: Stand straight and keep your left arm extended and thumbs up. Raise your arm, holding the weight at a 30-degree angle with your thumb up. Hold the position for a second then slowly return to your starting position.

Focus: Keeping your arm lifted at a right angle.

Feeling: You will feel this in the front of the rotator cuff

Key points: Keep your balance while holding the weight. Hold the weight in your finger tips.

Time or Reps: Complete 3 sets of 10 reps.

Difficulty level: 1 of 5

Shoulder Flexion Thumbs Down (Right Arm) - 5 Pounds 3 X 10

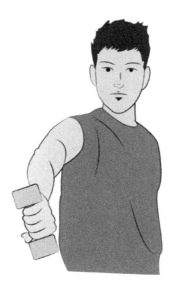

Instructions: Stand straight with your right arm extended and your thumb pointing down. Keeping the elbow straight, hold the weight at a 30 degree angle. Slowly move your arms in an upward direction. Hold this move at the top for a second then slowly lower the weight .

Focus: Your arm should be straight and at a 30 degree angle in front of the body with your thumb facing down.

Feeling: You should feel resistance on the top side of the posterior cuff

Key points: Keep your body straight and if you feel pain or any unfamiliar pain, do not do this exercise. Lift nothing greater than 5 pounds.

Time or Reps: Complete 3 sets of 10 reps.

Difficulty level: 2 of 5

Shoulder Flexion Thumbs Down (Left Arm) - 5 Pounds 3 X 10

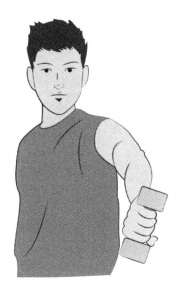

Instructions: Stand straight with your Left arm extended and thumb point down. Keeping the elbow straight, hold the weight an down your arms in an upwards direction. Slowly keep the movement and bring it back to the starting position.

Focus: Your arm should be straight with your thumb facing down.

Feeling: The movement of rotator cuff in an upward of the joint should be felt, as well as stretching in your biceps, triceps and clavicle.

Key points: Keep your body straight and if you feel pain or any unfamiliar pain, do not do this exercise. Lift nothing greater than 5 pounds.

Time or Reps: Complete 3 sets of 10 reps.

Difficulty level: 2 of 5

Shoulder Shrugs

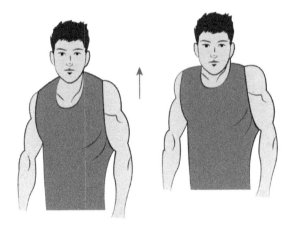

Instructions: Stand up straight. Now keep both arms steady on your side. Start moving your shoulders in an upward direction towards your ears. Slowly return to your position and repeat the process. This move requires heavy weight. Dumbbells preferred.

Focus: Keeping your back straight and your elbows a little flexed.

Feeling: You should feel this in your shoulder and traps.

Key points: Maintain good posture. Do not overdue the weight here. Add enough weight to feel some resistance.

Time or Reps: Complete 3 sets of 10 reps.

Difficulty level: 3 of 5

Sideling External Rotation (Right Arm) – 5 Pounds 3 X 10

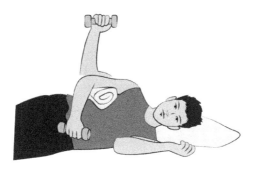

Instructions: Lay down on your left side keeping your right arm upwards. Place a towel or a rolled cloth under your right arm. Now bend your elbow at 90 degree angle. Externally rotate the weight lifting the weight. Slowly move your arm for the full range and then move your arm back down slowly. A 5 count on the way down will additionally benefit the shoulder.

Focus: Keep your elbow at a 90-degree. Do not lift your arm off the towel.

Feeling: You should feel rotation at your elbow joint. All the muscles in scapula including rotator cuff are initiated in this movement. This will help shoulder strength, durability and stability. You should feel a deep burn in the back of your shoulder.

Key points: Keep your arm at 90 degrees with a normal breathing pattern. Slowly lower the weight for 5 to 10 seconds each rep.

Time or Reps: Complete 3 sets of 10 reps.

Difficulty level: 2 of 5

Note - This is one of the preferred moves for shoulder injury recovery. Especially overhead athletes.

Sideling External Rotation (Left Arm) – 5 Pounds 3 X 10

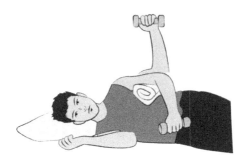

Instructions: Lay down on your right side keeping your left arm upwards. Place a towel or a rolled cloth under your left arm. Now bend your elbow at 90 degree angle. Externally rotate the weight lifting the weight. Slowly move your arm for the full range and then move your arm back down slowly. A 5 count on the way down will additionally benefit the shoulder.

Focus: Keep your elbow at a 90-degree. Do not lift your arm off the towel.

Feeling: You should feel rotation at your elbow joint. All the muscles in scapula including rotator cuff are initiated in this movement. This will help shoulder strength, durability and stability. You should feel a deep burn in the back of your shoulder.

Key points: Keep your arm at 90 degrees with a normal breathing pattern. Slowly lower the weight for 5 to 10 seconds each rep.

Time or Reps: Complete 3 sets of 10 reps.

Difficulty level: 2 of 5

Note - This is one of the preferred moves for shoulder injury recovery. Especially overhead athletes.

Sideling Internal Rotation (Right Arm) – 5 Pounds 3 X 10

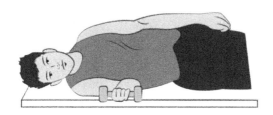

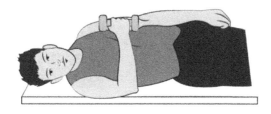

Instructions: Lay down over your right arm. Keeping arms on the side, bend your right arm at a 90-degree. Now slowly lift your hand using the elbow towards the internal side.

Focus: You should lie down on the involved side. Keeping your elbow at 90 degrees.

Feeling: You should feel resistance on the anterior side of the rotator cuff.

Key points: Move slowly and do not over rotate externally.

Time or Reps: Complete 3 sets of 10 reps.

Difficulty level: 2 of 5

Sideling Internal Rotation (Left Arm) – 5 Pounds 3 X 10

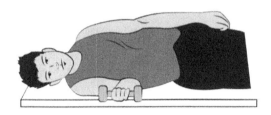

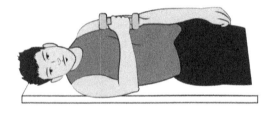

Instructions: Lie down over your left arm. Keeping arms on the side, bend your left arm at a 90-degree angle. Now slowly lift your hand using the elbow towards the internal side.

Focus: You should lie down on the involved side. Keep your elbow at 90 degrees.

Feeling: You should feel resistance on the anterior side of the rotator cuff.

Key points: Move slowly and do not over rotate externally.

Time or Reps: Complete 3 sets of 10 reps.

Difficulty level: 2 of 5

Horizontal Abduction

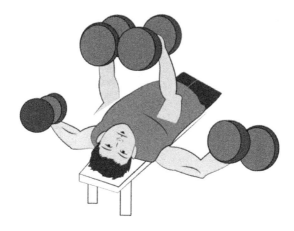

Instructions: Lay down on a bench on your back. Hold a light dumbbell in both hands. Extend your arms outward in a fly position. Now slowly lift your arms upwards until the fingers face the ceiling. Slowly move your arms and bring back to the starting position.

Focus: You should focus on slow movement and maintain a 90-degree angle.

Feeling: Resistance across your chest muscles and the front of your shoulder.

Key points: Keep your body straight and if you feel pain or any unfamiliar pain, don't do this exercise.

Time or Reps: Complete 3 sets of 10 reps.

Difficulty level: 4 of 5

Prone Flexion

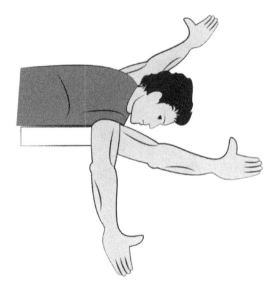

Instructions: Lie on a bench or table in a prone position. Keep your shoulders on the end on the table. Now lift your arms, pointing your thumbs upwards. Start moving your arms upwards slowly and extend them above your ears.

Focus: You should keep your arms straight. Get an extra flex at the top of the movement.

Feeling: You should feel movement of the shoulder in an upward direction. Resistance shoulder be felt in posterior cuff and scapula causing a slight burn on the back of your shoulder.

Key points: Keep your body straight and extend fully up. You should focus on holding the top of the movement.

Time or Reps: Complete 3 sets of 10 reps.

Difficulty level: 4 of 5

Prone Abduction

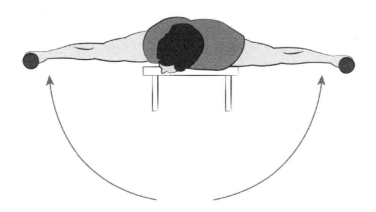

Instructions: Lay on a table in a prone position. Keep your shoulders on the end on the table. Drop your arms on the side of the tables; palms facing downwards or thumbs skyward. Then hold weights in both the hands in your finger tips. Slowly lift both arms upwards.

Focus: You should keep your arms straight and aligned with your shoulders.

Feeling: You should feel movement of the shoulder in a backwards direction. Movement of rotator cuff and scapula causing stretch in your arms, ribs cage and shoulder back.

Key points: Keep your body straight and if you feel pain or any unfamiliar pain, readjust your position. You don't need a table or bench, but it makes this moves easier.

Time or Reps: Complete 3 sets of 10 reps.

Difficulty level: 4 of 5

Prone Scapular Retraction with External Rotation

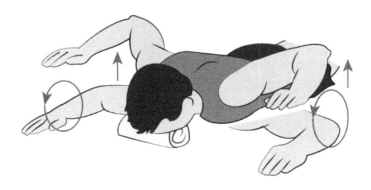

Instructions: Lay on a table in a prone position. Keep your shoulders on the end of the table. Drop your arms on the side of the table, palms facing downwards, and hold the weights (optional) in both the hands. Now slowly lift both arms in an upward direction. Firstly, bend your elbows at a 90-degree angle and then lift your arms in at shoulder level. This involves the movement of the elbow joint and the shoulder joint.

Focus: Load your scapula first, then bend your elbows and feel your posterior cuff lift the weights as you externally rotate. Your elbows will start off straight and end up at a 90-degree angle.

Feeling: You should feel a compound shoulder movement in a backwards direction, involving all your posterior shoulder muscles. Movement of the rotator cuff and scapula cause functional resistance for any shoulder using athlete.

Key points: Start with light weight and over time increase to 5 pounds.

Time or Reps: Complete 3 sets of 10 reps.

Difficulty level: 5 of 5

Arm to Side - External Rotation with Band - Right Arm

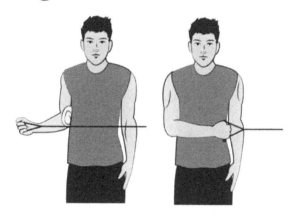

Instructions: Using a secure resistance band. The band should be tied at the elbow level. Stand on the right side of your band. Grab the end of the band with your right hand and press your elbow firmly to your side. The elbow should be at a 90-degree angle. Keep your hand in front of your torso. Start pulling the band in a external motion and keep your elbow level with the ground. Keep the movement smooth and stretch the band as far as you can externally rotate..

Focus: Slowly move the band and squeeze the movement at the top.

Feeling: You should feel resistance on the external muscles of your posterior cuff.

Key points: For maximum benefit place a rolled towel under your arm. This will keep separation needed for optimal rotator cuff strengthening.

Time or Reps: Complete 3 sets of 10 reps.

Difficulty level: 1 of 5

Arm to Side - External Rotation with Band - Left Arm

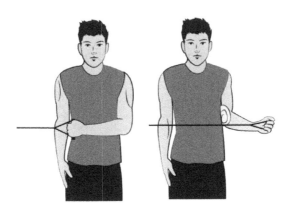

Instructions: Using a secure resistance band. The band should be tied at the elbow level. Stand on the left side of your band. Grab the end of the band with your left hand and press your elbow firmly to your side. The elbow should be at a 90-degree angle. Keep your hand in front of your torso. Start pulling the band in a external motion and keep your elbow level with the ground. Keep the movement smooth and stretch the band as far as you can externally rotate.

Focus: Slowly move the band and squeeze the movement at the top.

Feeling: You should feel resistance on the external muscles of your posterior cuff.

Key points: For maximum benefit place a rolled towel under your arm. This will keep separation needed for optimal rotator cuff strengthening.

Time or Reps: Complete 3 sets of 10 reps.

Difficulty level: 1 of 5

Arm to Side - Internal Rotation with Band - Right Arm

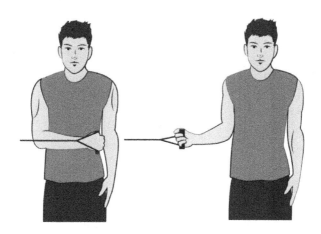

Instructions: Using a secure resistance band. The band should be tied at the elbow level. Stand on the left side of your band. Grab the end of the band with your right hand and press your elbow firmly to your side. The elbow should be at a 90-degree angle. Keep your hand in front of your torso. Start pulling the band in a internal motion and keep your elbow level with the ground. Keep the movement smooth and stretch the band as far as you can internally rotate.

Focus: Slowly move the band and squeeze the movement at the top.

Feeling: You should feel resistance on the anterior muscles of your rotator cuff.

Key points: The anterior side of the shoulder should be stronger then the posterior side

Time or Reps: Complete 3 sets of 10 reps.

Difficulty level: 1 of 5

Arm to Side - Internal Rotation with Band - Left Arm

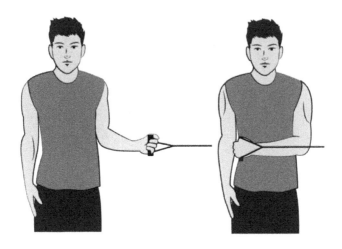

Instructions: Using a secure resistance band. The band should be tied at the elbow level. Stand on the right side of your band. Grab the end of the band with your left hand and press your elbow firmly to your side. The elbow should be at a 90-degree angle. Keep your hand in front of your torso. Start pulling the band in a internal motion and keep your elbow level with the ground. Keep the movement smooth and stretch the band as far as you can internally rotate.

Focus: Slowly move the band and squeeze the movement at the top.

Feeling: You should feel resistance on the anterior muscles of your rotator cuff.

Key points: The anterior side of the shoulder should be stronger then the posterior side

Time or Reps: Complete 3 sets of 10 reps.

Difficulty level: 1 of 5

Band Rows

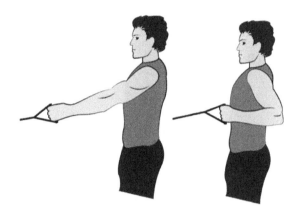

Instructions: Secure the resistance band. Grab the band with both hands. Start the move with the band at arm's length. Start pulling the band, pulling your arms behind and squeezing your elbows at a 90-degree angle. Pull and hold the position. Then slowly extend your arms.

Focus: Keep your back straight and squeeze your shoulders.

Feeling: You should feel resistance in the big back muscles. This move requires heavy resistance.

Key points: Keep your body straight move slow

Time or Reps: Complete 3 sets of 10 reps.

Difficulty level: 3 of 5

Lateral Deltoid Band Raise

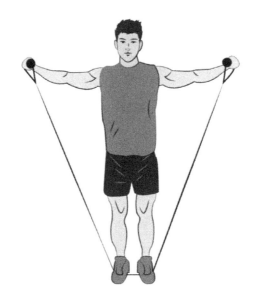

Instructions: Stand on the band so that tension is built when you raise the band at arm's length. Grab the ends of the band; the handles should be around your thighs. Bend your arms a little and keep your back straight. Use your shoulders to lift your hands until they are parallel to your shoulders. Keep your torso stationary and hold this position.

Focus: Keep your arms extended and parallel.

Feeling: Resistance should be felt in the rotator cuff and the top of the shoulder.

Key points: The angle of your arms shoulder be straight out from your shoulders.

Time or Reps: Complete 3 sets of 10 reps.

Difficulty level: 2 of 5

Bent Over Band Fly

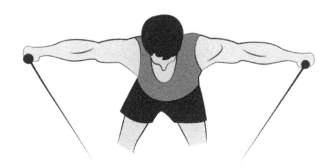

Instructions: Stand on the band so that tension is built at arm's length. Bend forward and keep your back straight. Grab the ends of the bands. The handles should be out front under your shoulders. Bend your body forward and your hips back. Keep your back straight. Now lift your arms upwards until they are parallel to your shoulders.

Focus: Keep your back straight and bend at the waist.

Feeling: You should feel resistance on your posterior cuff and scapula

Key points: Keep your back straight and flat. Keep your thumbs up or forward.

Time or Reps: Complete 3 sets of 10 reps.

Difficulty level: 2 of 5

Standing Shoulder Band Fly

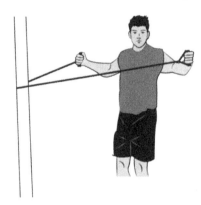

Instructions: Secure your resistance band around a pole (Our something secure). Face the pole, grab the handles of the band and step backward to increase the tension in the band. Bend your arms slightly at the elbow. Extend your hands outward level with your shoulders.

Focus: Keep your posture up and stretch your arms wide.

Feeling: You should feel resistance in your arms, back muscles and shoulders.

Key points: Move the band slowly. If you have to throw the band, step closer.

Time or Reps: Complete 3 sets of 10 reps.

Difficulty level: 2 of 5

Band Shoulder Extension – Right Arm

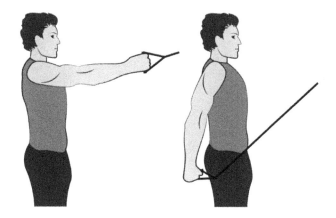

Instructions: Secure the band to a pole (or something secure). Facing towards the band. Stand straight and hold the band with your right arm. Keep your arm straight and extend the band down and backward behind to your hip.

Focus: Keep your arm and back straight. Squeeze the movement at the peak extension.

Feeling: You should feel resistance in your lat, posterior cuff and scapula.

Key points: Keep your body posture up. Step back if you need added resistance.

Time or Reps: Complete 3 sets of 10 reps.

Difficulty level: 2 of 5

Band Shoulder Extension – Left Arm

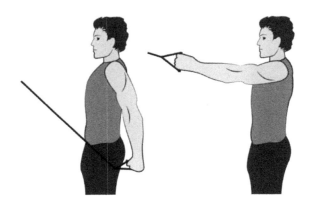

Instructions: Secure the band to a pole (or something secure). Facing towards the band. Stand straight and hold the band with your left arm. Keep your arm straight and extend the band down and backward behind to your hip.

Focus: Keep your arms and back straight. Squeeze the movement at the peak extension.

Feeling: You should feel resistance in your lat, posterior cuff and scapula.

Key points: Keep your body posture up. Step back if you need added resistance.

Time or Reps: Complete 3 sets of 10 reps.

Difficulty level: 2 of 5

Band Shoulder Diagonal Flexion - Right Arm

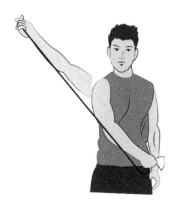

Instructions: Secure the band to a pole (or another secure location). Make sure the band is secure near the ground. The band should be slightly above ground to knee-length. Stand with your left shoulder facing towards the secured band. Hold the end of the band with your right arm. Extend the band in a diagonal direction up and outwards away from the opposite hip. Keep your arm straight during this move. Extension of your arm should reach slightly behind your head. Hold this position for a second, then slowly return to the starting position and repeat.

Focus: Your focus should be on keeping your arm straight and stretching full range of motion. Move slowly.

Feeling: You should feel resistance in your upper shoulder and posterior cuff.

Key points: Keep your body straight and move your arm across your body. Make sure your band can stretch far enough for full range.

Time or Reps: Complete 3 sets of 10 reps.

Difficulty level: 2 of 5

Band Shoulder Diagonal Flexion - Left Arm

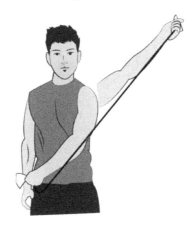

Instructions: Secure the band to a pole (or another secure location). Make sure the band is secure near the ground. The band should be slightly above ground to knee-length. Stand with your right shoulder facing towards the secured band. Hold the end of the band with your left arm. Extend the band in a diagonal direction up and outwards away from the opposite hip. Keep your arm straight during this move. Extension of your arm should reach slightly behind your head. Hold this position for a second, then slowly return to the starting position and repeat.

Focus: Your focus should be on keeping your arm straight and stretching full range of motion. Move slowly.

Feeling: You should feel resistance in your upper shoulder and posterior cuff.

Key points: Keep your body straight and move your arm across your body. Make sure your band can stretch far enough for full range.

Time or Reps: Complete 3 sets of 10 reps.

Difficulty level: 2 of 5

Band Shoulder Press Standing

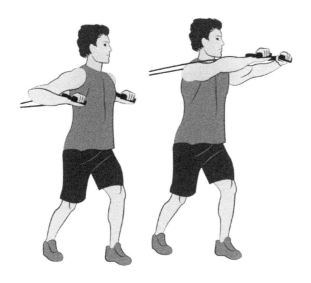

Instructions: Secure a band behind you. Hold both ends of the band with your hands. Lean forward with your feet apart. Keep your arms bent at the elbows and step forward until you feel slight resistance. Then use just your arms to push the band straight outward. Fully extend your arms forward then slowly return to the starting position.

Focus: Your focus should be on pressing the bands outward with your chest.

Feeling: You should feel resistance in your chest and front of your shoulder.

Key points: Step forward until the bands are fully extended. This move should require increased resistance.

Time or Reps: Complete 3 sets of 10 reps.

Difficulty level: 2 of 5

Band Chest Fly

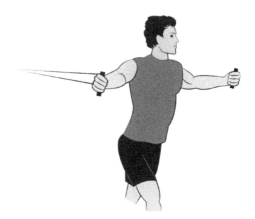

Instructions: Secure the band behind you. Lean forward with your feet apart. Keep your arms straight at your sides. Do not bend your elbows. Use your arms to extend the band in front of you at shoulder height. Resume this extended position for a second and then slowly return to the starting position.

Focus: Your focus should be on keeping your arms straight and using just your chest to extend the bands.

Feeling: You should feel resistance in your shoulder and chest.

Key points: Keep your posture up and only move your arms. Not your body.

Time or Reps: Complete 3 sets of 10 reps.

Difficulty level: 2 of 5

Band Bicep Curl

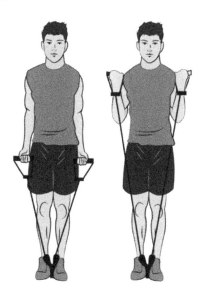

Instructions: Stand straight on the middle of a resistance band. Spread feet to increase the tension at arm's length. Hold the band with your pinky facing your thighs. Keep your back straight and slightly bend your elbow. Lift the band in an upward motion just using your biceps. Bring your hands to your shoulders. Squeeze at the top. Then slowly return to the original position.

Focus: Your focus should be on your biceps. Control the movement.

Feeling: You should feel resistance in your bicep and forearms.

Key points: Tighten your core and keep your posture straight.

Time or Reps: Complete 3 sets of 10 reps.

Difficulty level: 2 of 5

Band Tricep Pull-down

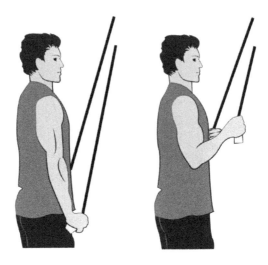

Instructions: Secure the band above your while facing the band. The end of the band should be about chest height. Hold both ends of the band and extend down until your arms are straight. Hold this position and then slowly return to your starting position.

Focus: Your focus should be on your triceps. Keep your back straight and your elbows close to your sides.

Feeling: You should feel resistance in your triceps.

Key points: If you need to bend over some, this is ok. Just try not to use your abs.

Time or Reps: Complete 3 sets of 10 reps.

Difficulty level: 2 of 5

Bands Scapular Loading

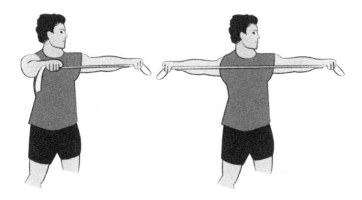

Instructions: Stand straight and keep your feet apart at hip length. Now hold the exercise band in your hands and extend it away from your torso at arm's length. Stretch the band in an outward direction. Stretch it until your arms are perpendicular to the ground. Hold this position and then slowly return to the starting position.

Focus: You focus should be on keeping your arms and your back straight.

Feeling: You should feel resistance in your scapula and torso

Key points: Focus on "loading" your scapula

Time or Reps: Complete 3 sets of 10 reps.

Difficulty level: 2 of 5

Lifted Arm External Rotation - Right Arm

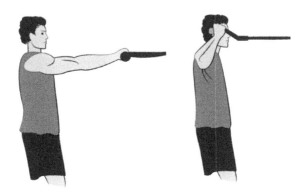

Instructions: Secure your band at shoulder height. Use your right hand to hold the band and step back as needed. Begin pulling the band backward with your scapula. Once your scapula is fully loaded, begin pulling back the band by bending your elbow. Keep your arm at shoulder height. Then begin to externally rotate your shoulder, lifting your hand backwards with your shoulder (see picture to the right).

Focus: Your arm shoulder fully complete each movement, on at a time, focusing on different muscles throughout the complex move. Then move onto the next movement.

Feeling: You should feel resistance in your back and your posterior cuff.

Key points: Form is important. Make sure your arm does not drop below shoulder height.

Time or Reps: Complete 3 sets of 10 reps.

Difficulty level: 3 of 5

Lifted Arm External Rotation - Left Arm

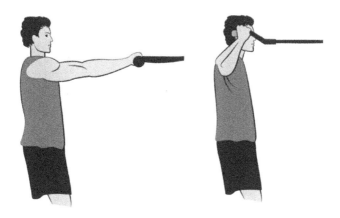

Instructions: Secure your band at shoulder height. Use your left hand to hold the band and step back as needed. Begin pulling the band backward with your scapula. Once your scapula is fully loaded, begin pulling back the band by bending your elbow. Keep your arm at shoulder height. Then begin to externally rotate your shoulder, lifting your hand backwards with your shoulder (see picture to the right).

Focus: Your arm shoulder fully complete each movement, on at a time, focusing on different muscles throughout the complex move. Then move onto the next movement.

Feeling: You should feel resistance in your back and your posterior cuff.

Key points: Form is important. Make sure your arm does not drop below shoulder height.

Time or Reps: Complete 3 sets of 10 reps.

Difficulty level: 3 of 5

Scapular Pushup

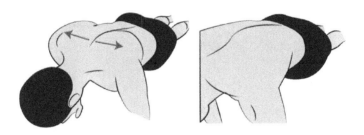

Instructions: Lie down on the floor, facing the ground with your arms apart, hands under shoulders. Hold your torso up in a push up position. Lift your body up and down while keeping your arms straight. This will require loading and unloading your scapula.

Focus: Keep your body straight and flat. Focus on your shoulders.

Feeling: There should be movement of your scapular muscles up and down.

Key points: Keep your arms straight. This is not a full push-up.

Time or Reps: Complete 3 sets of 10 reps.

Difficulty level: 2 of 5

Dog Pointers - Left Arm

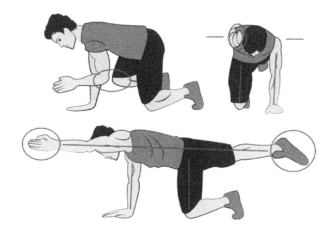

Instructions: Start with a four-point stance on the ground, on your hands and knees. Make sure the hips are at approximately 90-degrees. Start by stretching one leg outwards, keeping your hips leveled and extending the opposite arm out in front of you. Hold for about 2 seconds and then crunch your elbow and knee together. Then extend back out and repeat.

Focus: Achieve full extension and touch your elbow to your knee.

Feeling: You would feel resistance in the back of your shoulder and your core.

Key points: Hold your position and move slowly.

Time or Reps: Complete 3 sets of 10 reps

Difficulty level: 1 of 5

Dog Pointers - Right Arm

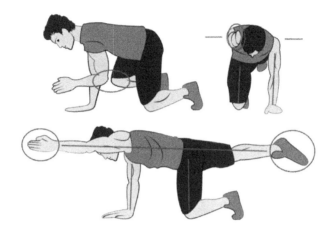

Instructions: Start with a four-point stance on the ground, on your hands and knees. Make sure the hips are at approximately 90-degrees. Start by stretching one leg outwards, keeping your hips level and extending the opposite arm out in front of you. Hold for about 2 seconds and then crunch your elbow and knee together. Then extend back out and repeat.

Focus: Achieve full extension and touch your elbow to your knee.

Feeling: You would feel resistance in the back of your shoulder and your core.

Key points: Hold your core position and move slowly.

Time or Reps: Complete 3 sets of 10 reps

Difficulty level: 1 of 5

Dog Pointer Lateral - Left Arm

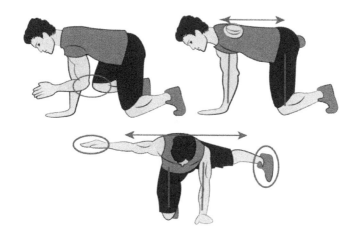

Instructions: Start with a four-point stance on your hands and knees. Make sure your hips at 90 degrees. Start by stretching one leg outwards laterally, keeping your hips level and extending the opposite arm out laterally. Hold for about 2 seconds and then crunch your elbow and knee together. Then extend back out and repeat.

Focus: Achieve full extension and touch your elbow to your knee.

Feeling: You would feel resistance in the back of your shoulder and your core.

Key points: Hold your core position and move slowly.

Time or Reps: Complete 3 sets of 10 reps

Difficulty level: 1 of 5

Dog Pointer Lateral - Right Arm

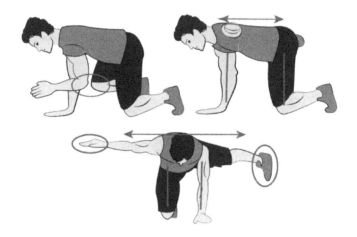

Instructions: Start with a four-point stance on your hands and knees. Make sure your hips at 90 degrees. Start by stretching one leg outwards laterally, keeping your hips level and extending the opposite arm out laterally. Hold for about 2 seconds and then crunch your elbow and knee together. Then extend back out and repeat.

Focus: Achieve full extension and touch your elbow to your knee.

Feeling: You would feel resistance in the back of your shoulder and your core.

Key points: Hold your core position and move slowly.

Time or Reps: Complete 3 sets of 10 reps

Difficulty level: 1 of 5

Side Plank Hold on Knees – Right Side

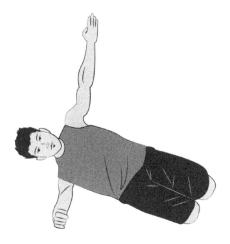

Instructions: Lie on your right side. Use a mat when necessary. Bend both knees and keep your legs together. Position your left arm perpendicularly above to your body (see the picture to the right). Bend your right elbow at a 90-degree angle. Now raise your upper body using the strength of your right arm and right oblique. Extend your left arm over your head. The left arm should be straight without any bend at the elbow. Hold this position.

Focus: Your focus should be on maintaining a straight spine position. Keep your elbow directly underneath your body.

Feeling: You should feel resistance in your core and stability in your shoulder.

Key points: Hold as still as possible.

Time or Reps: Hold for 30 seconds. As you gain strength progress to 60 seconds.

Difficulty level: 3 of 5

Side Plank Hold on Knees – Left Side

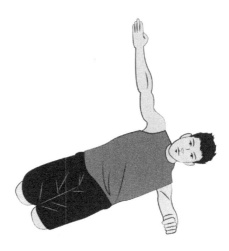

Instructions: Lie on your left side. Use a mat when necessary. Bend both knees and keep your legs together. Position your right arm perpendicularly above to your body (see the picture to the right). Bend your left elbow at a 90-degree angle. Now raise your upper body using the strength of your left arm and left oblique. Extend your right arm over your head. The right arm should be straight without any bend at the elbow. Hold this position.

Focus: Your focus should be on maintaining a straight spine position. Keep your elbow directly underneath your body.

Feeling: You should feel resistance in your core and stability in your shoulder.

Key points: Stretch your arm straight and keep your body in balance.

Time or Reps: Hold for 30 seconds. As you gain strength progress to 60 seconds.

Difficulty level: 3 of 5

Straight Arm Extended Side Plank Hold – Right Arm

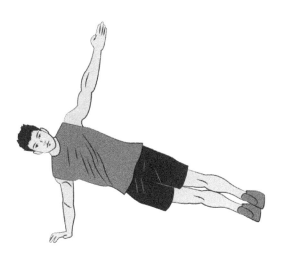

Instructions: Lie on your right side on an exercise mat. Raise your body by straightening your right arm underneath your shoulder. Extend both legs outward with feet stacked. Now extend your left arm in a straight position above your body. Hold this position.

Focus: Maintain your balance and keep your body straight.

Feeling: You should feel resistance in your core and stability in your shoulder.

Key points: Stretch your arm straight and keep your body in balance. Focus on your shoulder stability.

Time or Reps: Hold for 30 seconds. As you gain strength progress to 60 seconds.

Difficulty level: 4 of 5

Straight Arm Extended Side Plank Hold – Left Arm

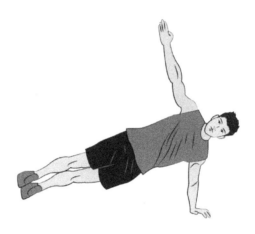

Instructions: Lie on your left side with an exercise mat. Raise your body by straightening your left arm underneath your shoulder. Extend both legs outward with feet stacked. Now extend your right arm in a straight position above your body. Hold this position.

Focus: Maintain your balance and keep your body straight.

Feeling: You should feel resistance in your core and stability in your shoulder.

Key points: Stretch your arm straight and keep your body in balance. Focus on your shoulder stability.

Time or Reps: Hold for 30 seconds. As you gain strength progress to 60 seconds.

Difficulty level: 4 of 5

Dumbbell Fly With Bent Arm Plank – Left Arm

Instructions: Lie on your right side on an exercise mat. Straighten your legs and keep them together. Stack your feet Bend your right elbow at a 90-degree angle under your shoulder while lifting the body. Now raise your upper body using the strength of your right arm. With a dumbbell 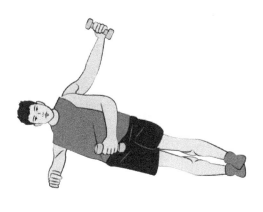 (5 lbs) in your left hand, extend your left arm over your head to hold the weight up. Your arm should be straight and should not bend at the elbow. Now slowly lower the weight in front of your body with your left arm still straight. Once you extend the dumbbell shoulder level in front of you, bring the weight back up to the starting position.

Focus: Your focus should be on maintaining a straight spine while you slowly lift the dumbbell.

Feeling: You should feel your core flex and the your down shoulder stabilizing the movement. The dumbbell arm should feel resistance in the posterior cuff and scapula.

Key points: Make sure the dumbbell is straight out front with your thumb down. Be careful on this move, it is advanced.

Time or Reps: Complete 3 sets of 10 reps.

Difficulty level: 5 of 5

Dumbbell Fly and With Bent Arm Plank – Right Arm

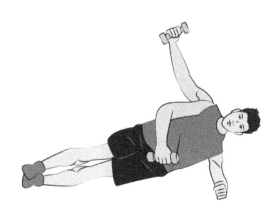

Instructions: Lie on your left side on an exercise mat. Straighten your legs and keep them together. Stack your feet Bend your left elbow at a 90-degree angle under your shoulder while lifting the body. Now raise your upper body using the strength of your left arm. With a dumbbell (5 lbs) in your right hand, extend your right arm over your head to hold the weight up. Your arm should be straight and should not bend at the elbow. Now slowly lower the weight in front of your body with your right arm still straight. Once you extend the dumbbell shoulder level in front of you, bring the weight back up to the starting position.

Focus: Your focus should be on maintaining a straight spine while you slowly lift the dumbbell.

Feeling: You should feel your core flex and the your down shoulder stabilizing the movement. The dumbbell arm should feel resistance in the posterior cuff and scapula.

Key points: Make sure the dumbbell is straight out front with your thumb down. Be careful on this move, it is advanced.

Time or Reps: Complete 3 sets of 10 reps.

Difficulty level: 5 of 5

Side Plank with Oblique Twist – Left Arm

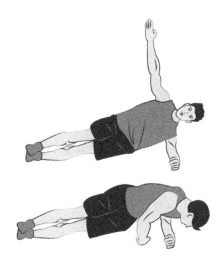

Instructions: Lie to your left side on an exercise mat. Now straighten your legs and stack them. Position your left arm under your shoulder. Bend your left elbow at a 90-degree angle. Raise your upper body using the strength of your left arm. Now extend your right arm upwards and keep it straight, and then rotate your arm and body internally towards your torso. Then take your hand reach under your body. Once you are at full range of motion, work backwards on the same path until your hand and torso are at your starting potion (see picture to the right).

Focus: Your focus should be on your down shoulder being stable and using your core to slowly move your body as you rotate.

Feeling: You should feel deep resistance in the shoulder and core. Stability in your rotator cuff will be tested here.

Key points: Move very slow and only do as many reps as you can handle with good form.

Time or Reps: Complete 3 sets of 10 reps.

Difficulty level: 4 of 5

Side Plank with Oblique Twist – Right Arm

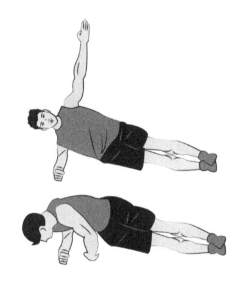

Instructions: Lie to your right side on an exercise mat. Now straighten your legs and stack them. Position your right arm under your shoulder. Bend your right elbow at a 90-degree angle. Raise your upper body using the strength of your right arm. Now extend your left arm upwards and keep it straight, and then rotate your arm and body internally towards your torso. Then take your hand reach under your body. Once you are at full range of motion, work backwards on the same path until your hand and torso are at your starting potion (see picture to the right).

Focus: Your focus should be on your down shoulder being stable and using your core to slowly move your body as you rotate.

Feeling: You should feel deep resistance in the shoulder and core. Stability in your rotator cuff will be tested here.

Key points: Move very slow and only do as many reps as you can handle with good form.

Time or Reps: Complete 3 sets of 10 reps.

Difficulty level: 4 of 5

Side Plank with Oblique Twist Right Arm + A Light Dumbbell (5 to 10 lbs)

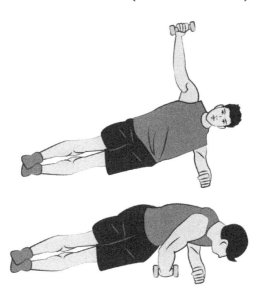

Instructions: Lie to your left side on an exercise mat. Now straighten your legs and stack them. Position your left arm under your shoulder. Bend your left elbow at a 90-degree angle. Raise your upper body using the strength of your left arm. Now extend your right arm upwards with a light dumbbell and keep it straight. Then rotate your arm and body internally towards your torso. Then take the dumbbell and reach under your body. Once you are at full range of motion, work backwards on the same path until your dumbbell and torso are at your starting potion (see picture to the right).

Focus: Your focus should be on your down shoulder being stable and using your core to slowly move your body as you rotate the dumbbell.

Feeling: You should feel deep resistance in the shoulder and core. Stability in your rotator cuff will be tested here.

Key points: Move very slow and only do as many reps as you can handle with good form. Only use a light dumbbell 5 to 10 pounds.

Time or Reps: Complete 3 sets of 5 to 10 reps.

Difficulty level: 5 of 5

Side Plank with Oblique Twist Left Arm + A Light Dumbbell (5 to 10 lbs)

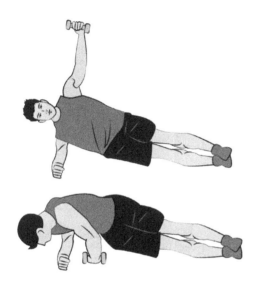

Instructions: Lie to your right side on an exercise mat. Now straighten your legs and stack them. Position your right arm under your shoulder. Bend your right elbow at a 90-degree angle. Raise your upper body using the strength of your right arm. Now extend your left arm upwards with a light dumbbell and keep it straight. Then rotate your arm and body internally towards your torso. Then take the dumbbell and reach under your body. Once you are at full range of motion, work backwards on the same path until your dumbbell and torso are at your starting potion (see picture to the right).

Focus: Your focus should be on your down shoulder being stable and using your core to slowly move your body as you rotate the dumbbell.

Feeling: You should feel deep resistance in the shoulder and core. Stability in your rotator cuff will be tested here.

Key points: Move very slow and only do as many reps as you can handle with good form. Only use a light dumbbell 5 to 10 pounds.

Time or Reps: Complete 3 sets of 5 to 10 reps.

Difficulty level: 5 of 5

Lateral Plank Hand Walking

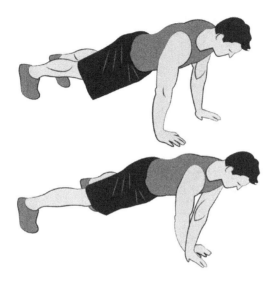

Instruction: Lie down in a plank position and place your hands underneath your shoulders. Simultaneously cross your right hand toward the left as you step your left foot out to the left side. Then step your left hand and right foot to the left, thus returning to the plank position. Your hands should move together as your feet step apart. Take two more steps in this direction while keeping your abs pulled towards your spine and your pelvis level.

Focus: Keep your back straight.

Feeling: You should feel resistance rotator cuff and in your deltoid.

Time or Reps: Make 5 movements to each side. Complete 3 sets

Difficulty level: 5 of 5

Dynamic Planks – Elbows to Hands

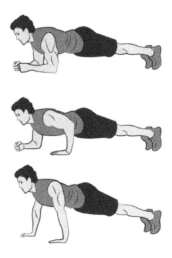

Instructions: Lie down on the floor, facing the ground and bending your arms at a 90–degree angle in front of your face. Hold your torso up with the help of your arms. Now use your hand to simultaneously lift your chest from the ground. Hold the position and slowly return back to your elbows. Then repeat the exercise.

Focus: Keep your body straight and do not slam your body down.

Feeling: You should feel intense resistance and stability in your shoulders.

Key points: When you regain your original position, hold for a while before you repeat the exercise. Be careful not to move to fast. This requires a significant amount of core strength.

Time or Reps: Complete 3 set of 5 to 10 reps.

Difficulty level: 5 of 5

External Weighted Ball Throws

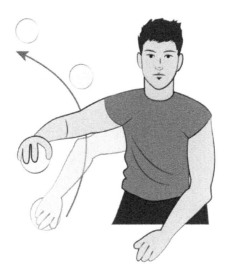

Instructions: Sit on a chair or stand near a wall. Hold a small medicine ball in your hand. Use the external rotation of your shoulder to throw the ball in an external motion. Move your arm from internal rotation to external rotation by throwing the ball backwards. Use a soft weighted ball (3 to 10 lbs) for this exercise. Throw the ball against a wall or with a partner.

Focus: Firmly grip the ball and start off with slow backward throws. Release the ball at max velocity backwards with your elbow high.

Feeling: You should feel resistance in your posterior cuff.

Time or Reps: Complete 10 throws. 3 sets.

Difficulty level: 4 of 5

Pull Ups Wide Grip

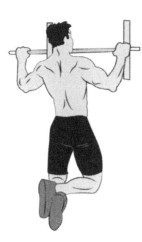

Instructions: Grab the bar with both arms parted wider than your shoulders. Lift your torso high enough so that your head rises above the bar. Then slowly return to the starting position.

Focus: Keep your grip and core tight through the movement

Feeling: When you lift your body, you should feel resistance in your lats and forearms.

Key points: Do not jerk your body up. Try to just use your lats to lift your body up.

Time or Reps: Complete 5 to 10 reps. 3 sets.

Difficulty level: 5 of 5

Pull-Ups Close Grips

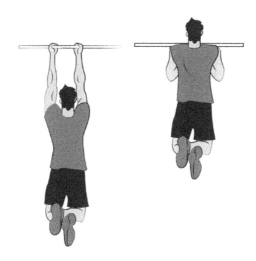

Instructions: Grab a bar with both arms at a close grip (1 to 2 inch separation) and palms back. Now lift your torso high enough that your head rises above the bar. Hold this position and then slowly return to the starting position.

Focus: Keep your elbows close to your body use your biceps to help pull you upward.

Feeling: When you lift your body, you should feel resistance in your lats and biceps.

Key points: Do not jerk your body up. Try to just use your lats to lift your body up.

Time or Reps: Complete 5 to 10 reps. 3 sets.

Difficulty level: 5 of 5

Physio Ball – Push Ups

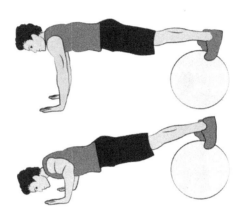

Instructions: Suspend your legs on an exercise ball and lean forwards, facing towards the ground. Keep your arms parallel to each other and maintain your balance. Keeping the pressure on the ball, begin doing slow push-ups. Push your chest closer to the ground and then lift your torso using your arm strength.

Focus: Keep your body straight over your hands and flex your core.

Feeling: You should feel deep contractions in your shoulder muscles, chest and core.

Key points: This move is more about stability than speed. Focus on slow movements and stability.

Time or Reps: Complete 5 to 10 reps. 3 sets.

Difficulty level: 5 of 5

Upright Row With Bar

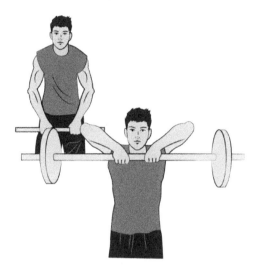

Instructions: Grab a barbell with an overhand grip. The bar should be leveled with your thighs and your arms should slightly bend at your elbows. Keep your back straight. Exhale and use your shoulders to lift the bar. Extend your elbows out and lift the bar until it reaches your chin. Inhale and lower the bar.

Focus: Your traps and shoulders should be driving the movement. Keep your posture straight.

Feeling: You should feel resistance in your shoulder and traps.

Key points: Do not throw the weight. Control the movement. Lower the weight if needed.

Time or Reps: Complete 3 sets of 10 reps.

Difficulty level: 5 of 5

Dumbbell Row Heavy – Right Arm

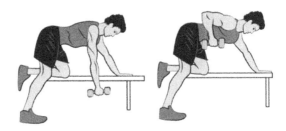

Instructions: Choose a flat bench and place your left hand on the bench. You have the option of placing your left leg on the bench as well. Bend your torso parallel to the floor. Use your right hand to lift up a heavy dumbbell from the floor. Pull the weight just below your chest. Keep your arms close to the side and your torso stationary. Keep your torso steady while you lift the weight.

Focus: You should be using heavy weight requiring you to use the big parts of your lat and deltoid.

Feeling: You should feel significant resistance in your back lat muscles and posterior shoulder.

Key points: Concentrate on squeezing your upper arm close to your side and lifting your elbow high without moving your torso.

Important: If you can complete your 3rd set and 10th rep with good form, you should go up in weight.

Time or Reps: Complete 3 to 4 sets of 10 reps.

Difficulty level: 5 of 5

Dumbbell Row Heavy – Left Arm

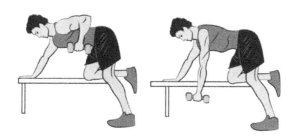

Instructions: Choose a flat bench and place your right hand on the bench. You have the option of placing your right leg on the bench as well. Bend your torso parallel to the floor. Use your left hand to lift up a heavy dumbbell from the floor. Pull the weight just below your chest. Keep your arms close to the side and your torso stationary. Keep your torso steady while you lift the weight.

Focus: You should be using heavy weight requiring you to use the big parts of your lat and deltoid.

Feeling: You should feel significant resistance in your back lat muscles and posterior shoulder.

Key points: Concentrate on squeezing your upper arm close to your side and lifting your elbow high without moving your torso.

Important: If you can complete your 3rd set and 10th rep with good form, you should go up in weight.

Time or Reps: Complete 3 to 4 sets of 10 reps.

Difficulty level: 5 of 5

Reverse Push Ups

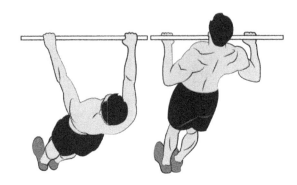

Instructions: Lower a barbell approximately 3 feet from the ground. Grab the bar with both arms at a wide separation length. Lift your torso high enough that your chest touches the bar. Keep your legs straight and use your shoulder muscles and back to lift your body. Hold this position and then slowly return to the starting position.

Focus: Keep your back straight and use your arms and shoulders to lift your torso.

Feeling: You should feel resistance in your back, biceps and shoulder muscles.

Key points: Keep your back straight. Exhale as you lift your body and inhale as you go back into your starting position. Flex your core to keep your body straight.

Time or Reps: Complete 3 sets of 10 reps.

Difficulty level: 5 of 5

Hand Wall Walk

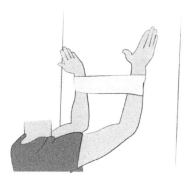

Instructions: Stand facing the wall. Place a circle connected band around both your wrists. Place your arms on the wall and bend them at a 90-degree angle. Now, slowly walk your hands up the wall while maintaining resistance in the band. Then walk your hands back down.

Focus: Focus on the distance between your hands. Maintain that separation as you walk your hands up and down.

Feeling: You should feel resistance in your posterior cuff.

Key points: Use a light band until your feel comfortable adding resistance. Keep your hand spread apart. As you fatigue, you will feel your hands move closer together. Do not allow this.

Time or Reps: Complete 3 sets of 10 reps.

Difficulty level: 3 of 5

Alternating Medicine Ball Push Ups

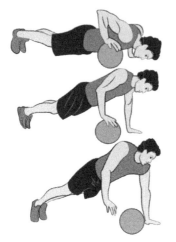

Instructions: Establish a push-up position with a firm medicine ball under your right hand. Place your other hand on the floor. Now start moving downwards and lower your chest to the ground. Extend upwards with the ball under your arm. Once you reach the top of the move, roll the ball to the other hand. Place your left hand on the ball and your right hand on the ground. Then complete another push-up. Repeat this process using alternative hands while you do push-ups.

Focus: Wrap a wide hand position around the medicine ball. Flex your core to help maintain balance

Feeling: This is a core exercise that includes the shoulders and chest. You will shake if you are weak. Be very careful. If your shoulder and chest are weak, you will not be able to do this.

Key points: This is an advanced move. If you have any shoulder injuries. Do not attempt this. Always move slowly on this move.

Time or Reps: Complete 3 sets of 10 reps (5 each arm)

Difficulty level: 5 of 5

Dual Medicine Ball Push Up

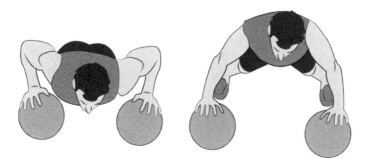

Instructions: Place two medicine balls underneath you. In a push-up position place your hands on each medicine ball. Start moving downwards and lower your chest close to the ground. During each push-up, slowly maintain balance.

Focus: You should be primarily focused on balance and stability. This is not a strength or reps move. It is a stability exercise.

Feeling: You will feel this in your shoulder, triceps, chest and core muscles.

Key points: Only do this move when you feel very good. Be very careful. Lower and raise your body slowly

Time or Reps: Complete 3 sets of 10 reps

Difficulty level: 5 of 5

Note: this move is only for the advanced.

Bench Plank Lateral Raise – Right Arm (5 to 10 lbs)

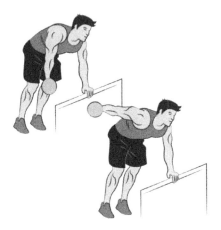

Instructions: Bend down on a bench with your left hand. Lift your right arm with a dumbbell laterally. While keeping your feet apart. Lift a weight in your right hand while keeping your arm straight. Bring your right arm in a perpendicular motion to the floor, hold the position at the top, and then move the dumbbell back down.

Focus: Keep your back straight. Keep your hand from falling back down.

Feeling: You should feel resistance in your posterior cuff and back muscles.

Key points: Lift the light dumbbell slowly.

Time or Reps: Complete 3 sets of 10 reps

Difficulty level: 5 of 5

Bench Plank Lateral Raise – Left Arm (5 to 10 lbs)

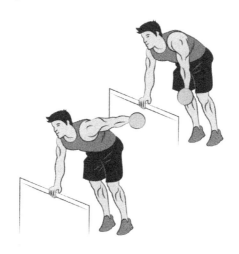

Instructions: Bend down on a bench with your right hand. Lift your left arm with a dumbbell laterally. While keeping your feet apart. Lift a weight in your left hand while keeping your arm straight. Lifting your left arm in a perpendicular motion to the floor, hold the position at the top, and then move the dumbbell back down.

Focus: Keep your back straight. Keep your hand from falling back down.

Feeling: You should feel resistance in your posterior cuff and back muscles.

Key points: Lift the light dumbbell slowly.

Time or Reps: Complete 3 sets of 10 reps

Difficulty level: 5 of 5

Dips

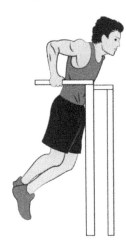

Instructions: Hold your dip bar with a firm grip. Keep your arms closer to your sides. Hold the bar and lift your body upwards with the support of your arms. Lean forewords and slowly push your body upwards. Then repeat

Focus: Keep your arms closer to your sides. Move slowly

Feeling: You will feel deep resistance in your shoulders and chest

Key points: This move is for strong healthy athletes.

Time or Reps: Complete 3 sets of 10 reps

Difficulty level: 5 of 5

CONCLUSION

I hope you enjoyed learning these workouts. A healthy shoulder takes time. Do not push yourself to quickly. I understand, everyone wants super fast progress. But you need to have a long term outlook on your rotator cuff. Slow progression leads to long term health. Trying to rush into advanced moves to quickly, can end up hurting you and slowing you down.

If you would like free videos explaining the most important rotator cuff exercises. Please click the link below:

www.RubberArmSeries.com

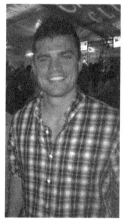

Many rotator cuff exercises are far easier to understand and execute by watching visual explanations of the exercise. That is why I created this website. I send out free videos to help my students achieve elite shoulder freedom. Plus you access to blueprints and plan to help you achieve your goals.

"Thanks for reading!" -Zach

Go ahead and visit rubberarmseries.com right now and subscribe with your email. You will get free videos of rotator cuff exercises and see with your own eyes, shoulder workouts and strategies for consistent long term health. I will see you there.

Click Below

www.RubberArmSeries.com

Made in the USA
Las Vegas, NV
06 April 2022